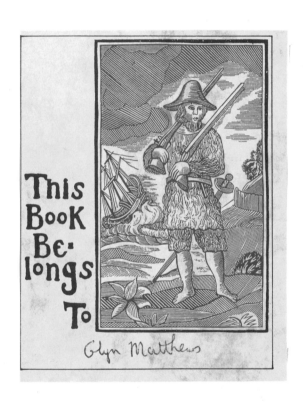

This Book Belongs To

Glyn Matthews

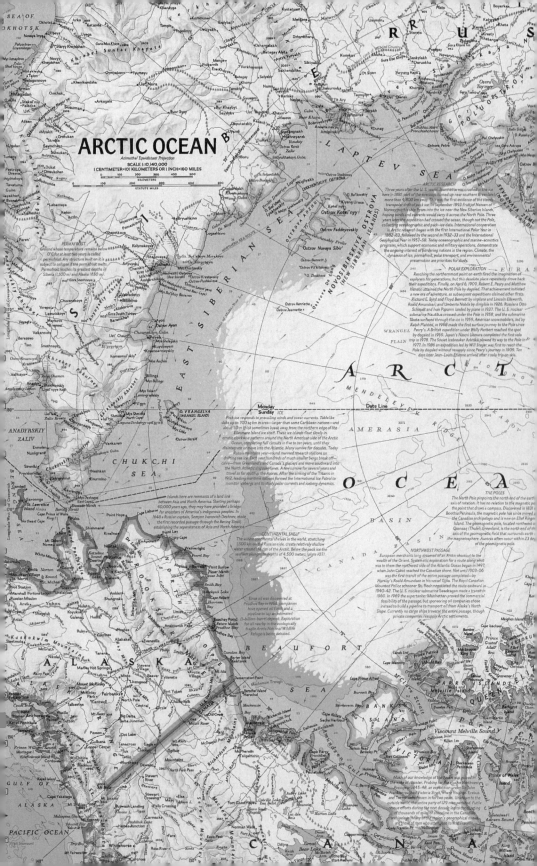

ARCTIC OCEAN

Azimuthal Equidistant Projection

SCALE 1:10,140,000
1 CENTIMETER=101 KILOMETERS OR 1 INCH=160 MILES

ARCTIC RESEARCH
Three years after the U.S. steamer *Jeannette* was crushed in the ice here in 1881, part of the wreckage turned up near southern Greenland more than 4,800 km away. This was the first evidence of the steady transpolar drift of pack ice. In September 1893 Fridtjof Nansen of Norway eased his ship frozen into the ice near the New Siberian Islands, hoping winds and currents would carry it across the North Pole. Three years later the expedition had crossed the ocean, though not the Pole, collecting oceanographic and pack-ice data. International cooperation in Arctic research began with the first International Polar Year in 1882–83, followed by the second in 1932–33 and the International Geophysical Year in 1957–58. Today oceanographic and marine-acoustics programs, which support economic and military operations, demonstrate the ongoing interest of bordering nations in the region. Climate, the dynamics of ice, permafrost, polar transport, and environmental preservation are priorities for study.

POLAR EXPLORATION
Reaching the northernmost point on earth fired the imagination of explorers for generations, but the desolate place repeatedly drove back their expeditions. Finally, on April 6, 1909, Robert E. Peary and Matthew Henson attained the North Pole by dogsled. That achievement initiated a new era of adventure, as subsequent expeditions claimed other firsts: Richard E. Byrd and Floyd Bennett by airplane and Lincoln Ellsworth, Roald Amundsen, and Umberto Nobile by dirigible in 1926. Russians Otto Schmidt and Ivan Papanin landed by plane in 1937. The U.S. nuclear submarine *Nautilus* crossed under the Pole in 1958, and the submarine *Skate* surfaced through the ice in 1959. American snowmobilers, led by Ralph Plaisted, in 1968 made the first surface journey to the Pole since Peary's. A British expedition under Wally Herbert reached the spot by dogsled in 1969. Japan's Naomi Uemura completed the first solo trip in 1978. The Soviet icebreaker *Arktika* plowed its way to the Pole in 1977. In 1986 an expedition led by Will Steger, was first to reach the Pole by dogsled without resupply since Peary's journey in 1909. Ten days later Jean-Louis Etienne arrived after a solo trip on ski.

ICE
Pack ice responds to prevailing winds and ocean currents. Tablelike slabs up to 700 sq km in area—larger than some Caribbean nations—and about 50 m thick sometimes break away from the northern edge of the Ellesmere Island ice shelf. These ice islands float slowly in erratic clockwise patterns around the North American side of the Arctic Ocean, completing full circuits in five to ten years, until they disintegrate or move into the Atlantic. Many survive for decades. Today Russia maintains year-round manned research stations on drifting sea ice. Each year hundreds of much smaller bergs break off—calve—from Greenland's and Canada's glaciers and move southward into the North Atlantic's shipping lanes. A few survive for several years and travel as far south as the Azores. After the sinking of the *Titanic* in 1912, leading maritime nations formed the International Ice Patrol to monitor icebergs and to study polar currents and iceberg dynamics.

CONTINENTAL SHELF
The widest continental shelves in the world, stretching 1,500 km on the Russian side, create relatively shallow water around the rim of the Arctic. Below the pack ice the sea floor plunges to depths of 4,500 meters (plate 107).

Since oil was discovered at Prudhoe Bay in 1968, companies have opened oil fields and a pipeline to tap an estimated 11-billion-barrel deposit. Exploration for oil nearby in the ecologically fragile Arctic National Wildlife Refuge is being debated.

Islands here are remnants of a land link between Asia and North America. Starting perhaps 40,000 years ago, they may have provided a bridge for ancestors of America's indigenous peoples. In 1648 a Russian captain, Semyon Ivanovich Dezhnev, made the first recorded passage through the Bering Strait, establishing the separateness of Asia and North America.

THE POLES
The North Pole pinpoints the north end of the earth's axis of rotation. It has no relation to the magnetic pole, the point that draws a compass. Discovered in 1831 on Boothia Peninsula, the magnetic pole has since moved off the Canadian archipelago and is now on Ellef Ringnes Island. The geomagnetic pole, located northwest of Qaanaaq (Thule), Greenland, is the north end of the axis of the geomagnetic field that surrounds earth's magnetosphere. Auroras often occur within 23 degrees of the geomagnetic pole.

NORTHWEST PASSAGE
European merchants long dreamed of an Arctic shortcut to the wealth of the Orient. Systematic exploration for a route along what was to become the northwest side of the Atlantic Ocean began in 1497, when John Cabot reached the Canadian shore. Not until 1903–06 was the first transit of the entire passage completed—by Norway's Roald Amundsen in his vessel *Gjöa*. The Royal Canadian Mounted Police schooner *St. Roch* negotiated the route eastward in 1940–42. The U.S. nuclear submarine *Seadragon* made a transit in 1960. In 1969 the supertanker *Manhattan* proved the commercial feasibility of the passage, but sponsoring oil companies chose instead to build a pipeline to transport oil from Alaska's North Slope. Currently no cargo ships traverse the entire passage, though private companies resupply Arctic settlements.

Much of our knowledge of the Arctic was gained amid scenes of disaster. Probing the maze of the Northwest Passage in 1845–48, an expedition under Sir John Franklin and his crew of 128 perished when their ships *Erebus* and *Terror* became frozen in the ice near King William Island. Franklin's own death, along with the outside world, the entire party of 129 men perished. Futile rescue efforts during the next decade led to the charting of thousands of miles of shoreline in the Canadian Arctic. Not until many years later was a geographical search at last found of one man who attempted to find Franklin.

PERMAFROST
Ground whose temperature remains below 0°C for at least two years is called permafrost. Any structure built on it is subject to collapse if the permafrost melts. Permafrost reaches its greatest depths in Siberia (1,500 m) and Alaska (650 m).

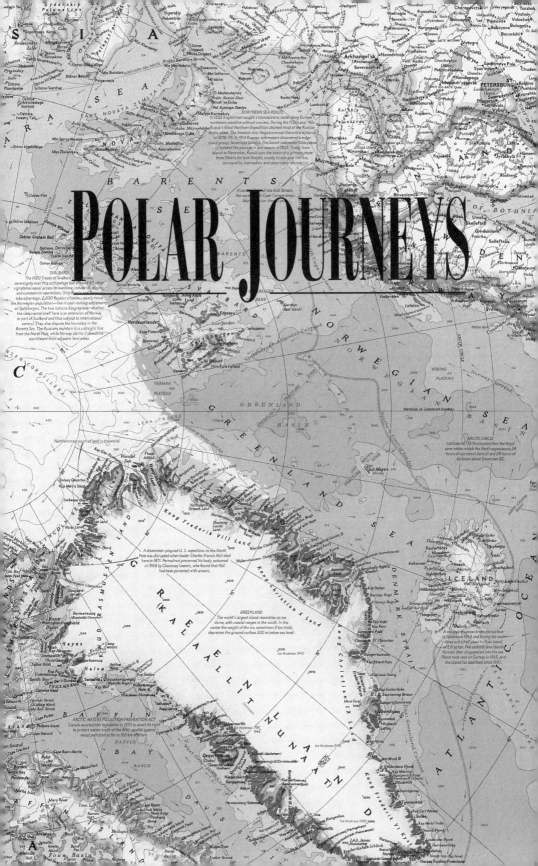

POLAR JOURNEYS

NORTHERN SEA ROUTE
In 1553 Englishmen sought a transoceanic route along Europe's northeast coastline without success. During the 1730s and '40s Russia's Great Northern Expedition charted most of the Russian Arctic coast. The Swedish ship Vega traversed the entire distance in 1878–79. In 1913 Russian icebreakers discovered a major island group, Severnaya Zemlya. The Soviet icebreaker Sibiryakov completed the passage in one season in 1932. Today, from March to November, Russia uses the ocean as a primary route from Siberia for bulk freight, mostly timber and iron ore, conveyed by icebreakers and observation planes.

A curling arm of the Gulf Stream, the warm North Cape Current keeps Murmansk ice-free.

SVALBARD
The 1920 Treaty of Svalbard gave Norway sovereignty over this archipelago but allowed 40 other signatories equal access to maritime, industrial, mining, and commercial operations. Only Russia and Norway take advantage; 2,200 Russian citizens—nearly twice the Norwegian population—live in coal-mining settlements on Spitsbergen. The two nations disagree over whether the continental shelf here is an extension of Norway or part of Svalbard and thus subject to international control. They also dispute the boundary in the Barents Sea. The Russians maintain it is a straight line from the North Pole, while Norway claims it be equidistant from adjacent land areas.

Northernmost point of land in the world.

ARCTIC CIRCLE
Latitude 66°33'N circumscribes the frigid zone within which the North experiences 24 hours of sun about June 21 and 24 hours of darkness about December 22.

A dissension-plagued U. S. expedition to the North Pole was disrupted when leader Charles Francis Hall died here in 1871. Permafrost preserved his body; exhumed in 1968 by Chauncey Loomis, who found that Hall had been poisoned with arsenic.

GREENLAND
The world's largest island resembles an ice dome, with coastal ranges in the south. In the center the weight of the ice, sometimes 3 km thick, depresses the ground surface 300 m below sea level.

A volcanic eruption broke the surface in November 1963 and during the next three and a half years built an island of 2.6 sq km. Two satellite lava islands formed, then disappeared into the sea. Plants took root on Surtsey in 1965, and the island has stabilized since 1967.

ARCTIC WATERS POLLUTION PREVENTION ACT
Canada enacted this legislation in 1970 to assert its right to protect waters north of the 60th parallel against vessel pollution as far as 160 km offshore.

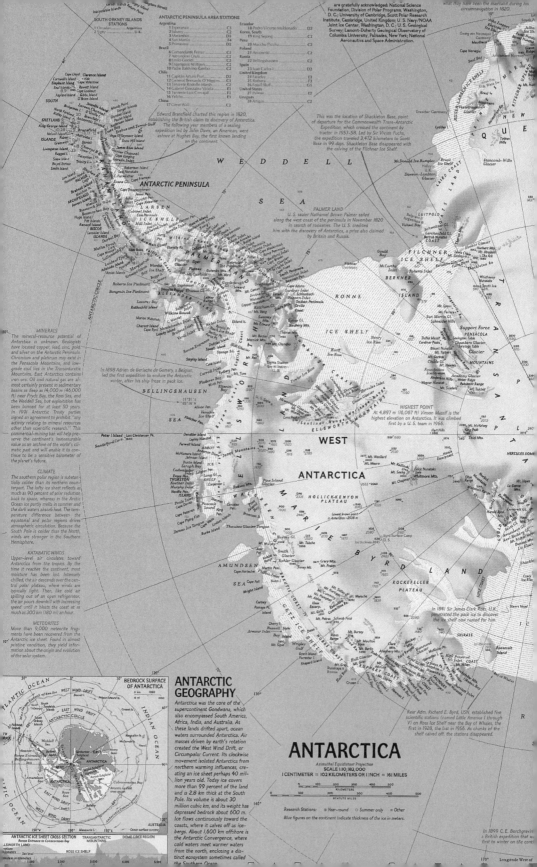

ANTARCTICA

Azimuthal Equidistant Projection
SCALE 1:10,182,000
1 CENTIMETER = 102 KILOMETERS OR 1 INCH = 161 MILES

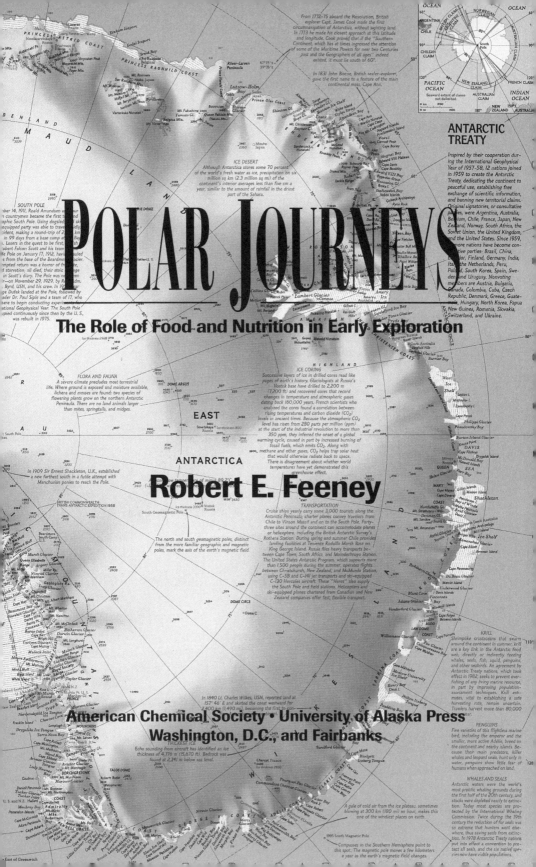

POLAR JOURNEYS

The Role of Food and Nutrition in Early Exploration

Robert E. Feeney

American Chemical Society • University of Alaska Press
Washington, D.C., and Fairbanks

Library of Congress Cataloging-in-Publication Data

Feeney, Robert Earl.
    Polar journeys : the role of food and nutrition in early
exploration / Robert E. Feeney.
        p.   cm.
    Includes bibliographical references and index.
    ISBN 0-8412-3349-7 (alk. paper). -- ISBN 0-912006-97-8 (pbk. :
alk. paper)
    1. Food--Preservation--History. 2. Nutrition--History. 3. Polar
regions--Discovery and exploration--History.   I. Title.
TX601.F44   1998   97-49810
641.4'09--dc21   CIP

International Standard Book Number: cloth, 0-8412-3349-7
                                                          paper, 0-912006-97-8
Library of Congress Catalogue Number: 97-49810

Printed in the United States by Thomson Shore, Inc.

This publication was printed on acid-free paper that meets the minimum
requirements of the American National Standards for Information Sciences-
Permanence of Paper for Printed Library Materials, ANSI Z39.48-1984.

Publication coordination by Pamela Odom of the University of Alaska Press
and Barbara Pralle and Cheryl Shanks of the American Chemical Society.

Publication, production, and cover design by Dixon J. Jones, Rasmuson
Library Graphics, University of Alaska Fairbanks.

American Chemical Society   University of Alaska Press
1155 Sixteenth Street, N.W.   1st Floor Gruening Building
Washington, DC 20036   P.O. Box 756240
(800) 227-5558   Fairbanks, Alaska 99775
                                   (907) 474-5831

The maps of the Arctic Ocean (pages ii–iii) and of Antarctica (pages iv–v)
are from the sixth revised edition of the *National Geographic Atlas*, courtesy
of the National Geographic Society.

To Mary Alice, my wife, who lovingly helped and supported me throughout my prolonged activity in this avocation

contents

illustrations

tables

preface

Like the origins of many books, the origins of this book had several different sources. At first glance, certainly, the sources would appear not only diverse but unrelated. However, they have all led me to a very deep respect for the role of food and nutrition in the lives of every living creature, from wild animals to polar explorers.

My first interest in foods, other than to supply my daily needs, was forced upon me during the depression of the 1930s while an undergraduate student in chemistry at Northwestern University in Evanston, Illinois. Here, I was lucky to obtain a job working for the Borden Company. While in and out of school, I held many different jobs with Borden, ranging from rising before dawn to deliver milk to lecturing on nutrition at clubs. While obtaining my doctoral degree in biochemistry at the University of Wisconsin, I was exposed to what was then one of the meccas of vitamin discoveries. Next, on my first post-Ph.D. job at Harvard Medical School, I was interested in nutrition but now searching for nutrients for microorganisms, not people. This led to my being commissioned in the U.S. Army in World War II as a food and nutrition officer in the Medical Department. Returning from the army, I again studied nutrients for microorganisms in the biochemistry department of a large government laboratory. But one morning on coming to my laboratory I found that the biochemistry department had been abolished and I had been placed in charge of a group to study the chemistry of eggs—back to human foods again. Then, after a stint as professor of chemistry at the University of Nebraska in Lincoln, I joined the Department of Food Science and Technology at the University of California in Davis as a biochemist.

Another source of this book lies in an accidental discovery. When I asked the U.S. Navy for some help in obtaining penguin eggs (for work on using evidence from evolution as a way to understand how enzymes and proteins work), the navy referred my request to the National Science Foundation (NSF), which handles all research and procurement of materials in Antarctica. Officials at NSF told me that I would have to go to Antarctica to get the penguin eggs myself. At first I did not want to go because the time required seemed unlikely to justify the results. Fortunately, however, I acquiesced to NSF, and I was exposed to a whole new vista and subsequently to a long and still continuing series of polar experiences. Many of these have been published in a short, older book, *Professor on the Ice*. Since 1964, I have participated in six separate research trips to Antarctica, going alone once, and at other times having as many as six students and coworkers with me. My antarctic work then led to an even greater number of similar trips with the Norwegians on their research ships, going from off the edge of the Russian island of Novaya Zemyla over to the northern ends of Spitsbergen (Svalbard) up in the arctic seas, to Newfoundland, to Alaska, and to the northern tip of Japan, where the Siberian currents come down in the wintertime. Thus, I have personally made over a dozen such trips. Six more were made by students and coworkers in my group, bringing my participation in or association with antarctic and arctic research trips to a total of twenty.

As a consequence of these trips, as well as many others in this country, Japan, and Europe, I have had the good fortune to meet and talk with many of the men involved in explorations from the early 1900s on through the 1950s. These included meeting on several occasions with the eminent Sir Charles Wright, who was a geologist associated with Robert Falcon Scott and who was with the group that discovered Scott and his companions frozen in their tent in 1912. (As a prelude to my first trip to Antarctica in 1964, I attended a planning session at Shenandoah National Park. There I slipped off a trail and was plucked up out of the mud by Sir Charles Wright. What an ignominious beginning.) Also, so many of those with Richard Byrd's group helped shape my interests and added to my knowledge, in either casual meetings or in prolonged talks, that it is hard to give them proper credit here, but to them all I owe a great debt. Recounting their many colorful chronicles would require a separate book. Standing out among these were Thomas Poulter, who had been the physicist leading the team that rescued Byrd from his toxic isolation episode, and Lawrence Gould, the geologist with Byrd. My many lucky contacts with polar people did not end with Byrd's group. While on a sabbatical at the Scott Polar Research Institute at Cambridge, I met Tryggbe Gran, the Norwegian who was associated with Scott, and the British Trans Antarctic Expedition leader and mountain climber, Sir Edmund Hillary.

Other sources of this book come from the publications on polar explorations I have read and collected—the latter certainly as a poor man's library. My interest in nutrition, combined with my fascination with polar exploration, led me to write this book. It has been impressed upon me how critical food and nutrition were to all of these explorers and their explorations. The knowledge of the times in the sciences of nutrition and food technology strongly influenced the explorers, while the needs of the explorations strongly influenced the developments in nutrition and food technology. Frequently the explorers were at the mercy of such decisions. Thus, the roots of the story lie in a mixture of science, technology, and the actions of people.

Some of the deeper roots lie in the decisions of people that caused immense suffering and death. Although most of these occurred nearly a century ago, or much earlier, and are remote from our thinking today, one in early California—the tragedy of the Donner Party—is easily comprehended. The party members died as a result of a bad decision to follow a poor route over the mountains late in the autumn, abetted by ignorance of ways to survive in the cold and snow. They apparently even might have survived had they known how to fish through the ice.

Over a twenty-year period I have read, and in some cases, perhaps half, I have reread the books and articles on the subjects in the bibliography. Initially a hobby, this study later became a major project. I am deeply appreciative and thankful to the many authors; what I have done is merely to assemble their materials in a way that expresses my opinions. I hope my opinions have not blurred the truth. Certainly, I have only included a very small fraction of the many reports and descriptions in the literature of polar exploration.

acknowledgments

I am indebted to so many individuals that I could not possibly list them all. So many have helped me by way of casual discussions that I cannot even remember all the sources. Colleagues and I had many discussions at night in quarters, sometimes while we lay in our sleeping bags, others while we were working in fish houses, flying in helicopters or airplanes, trekking through the snow, or just encountering one another any place around the earth.

I acknowledge particularly the more than thirty individuals who worked with me on my polar trips throughout the nearly twenty-five years of this continuing work.

I must acknowledge the gracious hospitality of the Norwegians, the Newfoundlanders, the Alaskans, and the Japanese and, of course, the excellent help of the U.S. National Science Foundation and the U.S. Navy in much of the work, particularly in Antarctica.

In writing this book I received extensive assistance in the supply of information from: Scott Polar Research Institute, Cambridge, England; Division of Polar Programs, National Science Foundation; U.S. National Aeronautics and Space Administration, Houston, Texas; U.S. Army Research Institute of Environmental Medicine, Natick, Massachusetts; University of Alaska Fairbanks; University of Saskatchewan; the University of California system; and libraries in Washington, D.C. The D.C. libraries were searched during two separate full weeks under a grant from the University of California, and included the National Archives, the Library of Congress, the National Library of Medicine, the Navy Historical Center, the Navy Medical Research Institute, and the National Geographic Society. Appreciation is particularly due to Dr. Albert Harrison, professor of psychology, University of California, Davis, and to Captain Brian Shoemaker, U.S. Navy, retired and former commander, McMurdo Station,

Antarctica; both not only critically read initial drafts but also supplied important comments in regard to their respective fields.

Nothing would have progressed without the fine secretarial assistance of several individuals. Ms. Chris Howland was the primary helper in the very early stages of the manuscript as well as related papers. Ms. Clara Robison successfully converted early material from an in-house computer program to a different format.

Some stand out particularly for their indirect help. Most important are my wife, Mary Alice, and my two daughters, Jane and Elizabeth, who supported my many and extensive trips to the far south or north, when often they didn't hear from me for weeks or even months.

chronology
Major Events in Exploration

c. 500   Brenden the Bold: Newfoundland or Nova Scotia (legend).

c. 1000 Erik the Red (Leif Erikson): Greenland, Labrador.

1576   Frobisher, Sir Martin: Shetlands, South Greenland, Frobisher Bay, Butchers Island.

1577   Frobisher, Sir Martin: Orkneys, Greenland, Baffin Island.

1578   Frobisher, Sir Martin: Canadian Arctic, Hudson Strait.

1585   Davis, John: South Greenland, Gilbert Sound, and Davis Strait.

1586   Davis, John: Greenland, Cumberland Sound, Hudson Bay, Hamilton Sound.

1587   Davis, John: West Greenland to Hope Sanderson.

1591   Davis, John: Falkland Islands; with Cavendish to 1593.

1594   Barents, Willem: Novaya Zemlya, Orange Islands, Vaigach Island.

1595   Barents, Willem: Vaigach Island, Kara Sea.

1596   Barents, Willem: Bear Island, Spitsbergen, Kola Peninsula.

1601   Davis, John: Table Bay, Cape of Good Hope to Madagascar, Chagos Archipelago, Nicobar Islands to Moluccas.

1607   Hudson, Henry: East Greenland, Spitsbergen.

1608   Hudson, Henry: Northeast Passage between Spitsbergen and Novaya Zemlya.

1609   Hudson, Henry: Barents Sea, Cape Cod, Hudson River.

1610   Hudson, Henry: Greenland, Hudson Strait and Bay, James Bay.

1612   Baffin, William: Greenland.

1613   Baffin, William: Spitsbergen.

1614   Baffin, William: Spitsbergen.

1615   Baffin, William: Hudson Strait to Southampton Island.

1616   Baffin, William: West Greenland to Smith Sound, Baffin Bay, Lancaster Sound.

1620   Baffin, William: Persian Gulf.

1724   Bering, Vitus: Kamchatka Peninsula, East Cape, Bering Strait.

1733   Bering, Vitus: Eastern Siberia.

1740   Bering, Vitus: Kayak Island, Alaska coast, Aleutians.

1759   Cook, James: St. Lawrence.

1768   Cook, James: Cape Horn, Tahiti, Society Islands, New Zealand, North Island, Cook Strait, South Island, Australia, Endeavor River, Torres Strait to Timor, Java, Strait of Sunda to Batavia.

1770   Hearne, Samuel: Hudson Bay, Chesterfield Inlet, Dubawnt Lake, Clinton Lake, Coppermine River, Great Slave Lake.

1772   Cook, James: Antarctica, New Zealand, Drake Strait (Drake Passage).

1774   Hearne, Samuel: Saskatchewan.

1776   Cook, James: Cape of Good Hope, Kerguelen Island, New Zealand, Sandwich Islands, Alaska, Bering Strait, coast of Asia.

1779   Mackenzie, Sir Alexander: Canada.

1785   Mackenzie, Sir Alexander: Lake Athabaska.

1789   Mackenzie, Sir Alexander: Slave River, Great Slave Lake, Mackenzie River.

1792   Mackenzie, Sir Alexander: Peace River, Parsnip Stream, Fraser River, Bella Coola River, Queen Charlotte Sound.

1806   Scoresby, William: East Greenland, Spitsbergen.

1818   Scoresby, William: Spitsbergen.

        Ross, Sir John: Baffin Bay, Ellesmere Land, Devon Island, Lancaster Sound.

        Ross, Sir James C.: Baffin Bay, Lancaster Sound.

        Parry, Lt. Sir William Edward: Baffin Bay, Lancaster Sound with J. Ross and J. C. Ross.

        Franklin, Sir John: north of Spitsbergen with Back.

        Back, Sir George: north of Spitsbergen with Franklin.

1819   Parry, Lt. Sir William Edward: Lancaster Sound, Melville Island with J. C. Ross.

        Franklin, Sir John: Hudson Bay, Great Slave Lake, Coppermine River, Cape Turnagain, with Back.

        Back, Sir George: Great Slave Lake, Coppermine River, with Franklin.

        Bellingshausen, Fabian Von: Rio de Janeiro, South Georgia, Antarctica, Alexander I Island, Australia.

        Ross, Sir James C.: Lancaster Sound, Barrow Strait with Parry.

1821   Ross, Sir James C.: Hudson Bay, with Parry.
        Parry, Lt. Sir William Edward/Fury and Hecla Strait.

1822   Scoresby, William: charted 200 miles north of Scoresby Sound on east coast of Greenland.

1824   Ross, Sir James C.: Lancaster Sound with Parry.

Parry, Lt. Sir William Edward/Lancaster Sound, Prince Regent Inlet with Ross.

1825   Franklin, Sir John: Mackenzie River, Point Barrow with Sir George Back.

Back, Sir George: Great Slave Lake, Mackenzie River, Great Bear Lake with Franklin.

1827   Parry, Lt. Sir William Edward: attempted North Pole.

1829   Ross, Sir James C.: King William Island.

Ross, Sir John: Canadian Arctic, Lancaster Sound, Prince Regent Inlet, Gulf of Boothia, King William Island.

1833   Back, Sir George: Great Slave Lake, Great Fish River, Cape Richardson, search expedition for Ross.

1836   Back, Sir George: Hudson Bay with ship *Terror*.

1839   Wilkes, Charles: east Antarctica, Wilkes Land, Tahiti, Samoas, Australia, New Zealand, Tonga Islands, Fiji, Sandwich Islands, Columbia River, Willamette, Sacramento River, Manila.

1840   Ross, Sir James C.: Antarctica, Ross Sea, Tasmania, Weddell Sea.

1845   Franklin, Sir John: Lancaster Sound, Somerset Island, Prince of Wales Island.

1846   Rae, Dr. John: Repulse Bay to Committee Bay.

1847   Rae, Dr. John: Committee Bay.

1848   Ross, Sir James C.: Canadian Arctic search for Franklin.

McClintock, Sir Francis Leopold: Search for Franklin, Baffin Bay with J.C. Ross.

1850   Ross, Sir John: Canadian Arctic search for Franklin.

McClintock, Sir Francis Leopold: Canadian Arctic, Cornwallis Island, Melville Peninsula.

1851   Rae, Dr. John: Search for Franklin, Coppermine River via Great Slave Lake and Great Bear Lake, Wollaston Land, Victoria Island.

1852   McClintock, Sir Francis Leopold: around Melville Island, Prince Patrick Island, search for Franklin.

Nares, Sir George Strong: Canadian Arctic search for Franklin, Lancaster Sound, Devon Island.

1854   Rae, Dr. John: Boothia Peninsula, east coast Kind William Island.

1857   McClintock, Sir Francis Leopold: Canadian Arctic, Boothia Peninsula, King William Island, Prince of Wales Island, McClintock Channel, found message left by Franklin.

1858   Nordenskjold, Baron Nils Adolf Erik: Went to Spitsbergen.

1861   Nordenskjold, Baron Nils Adolf Erik: attempted North Pole by dog sled.

1864   Nordenskjold, Baron Nils Adolf Erik: Spitsbergen.

1868   Nordenskjold, Baron Nils Adolf Erik: Spitsbergen.

1870   Nordenskjold, Baron Nils Adolf Erik: Greenland, Disko Island.

1872   Nares, Sir George Strong: command British Naval Expedition on Challenger, crossed Atlantic three times, via Capetown to Melbourne, New Zealand, East Indies, Japan, Sandwich Islands, Tahiti, Chile, Strait of Magellan to Montevideo, Ascension Island, to Azores.

       Nordenskjold, Baron Nils Adolf Erik: Phipps Island, Spitsbergen.

1875   Nordenskjold, Baron Nils Adolf Erik: Novaya Zemlya search for northeast passage to East.

1876   Nares, Sir George Strong: Canadian Arctic, Smith Sound, discovered the Challenger Mountains.

       Nordenskjold, Baron Nils Adolf Erik: second attempt to find northeast passage, Yenisei River.

1878   Nordenskjold, Baron Nils Adolf Erik: Discovered northeast passage along arctic coast of Asia, Bering Strait of Japan, returned to Scandinavia via new Suez Canal.

1879   De Long, George Washington: Bering Strait, ship marooned.

1882   Nansen, Fridtjof: East Greenland.

       First International Polar Year (forerunner of International Geophysical Year)

1883   Nordenskjold, Baron Nils Adolf Erik: second expedition to Greenland, Disko Island.

1886   Peary, Robert Edwin: Greenland exploration.

1888   Nansen, Fridtjof: South Greenland, Godthaab.

1891   Peary, Robert Edwin: Inglefield Gulf, Smith Sound, Independence Fiord, proved Greenland an island.

1893   Nansen, Fridtjof: Norway in the Fram, New Siberian Islands, North Pole attempt on foot unsuccessful, Franz Josef Land.

       Peary, Robert Edwin: Independence Fiord.

1898   Peary, Robert Edwin: Grant Land (Ellesmere Land), reached most northern part of Greenland.

1901   Scott, Robert Falcon: Antarctica expedition with Shackleton and Wilson, Cape Adare, discovered King Edward VII Land, proved Mt. Erebus and Mt. Terror on Ross Island, proved McMurdo Bay was a strait.

       Shackleton, Ernest Henry: Ross Barrier and King Edward VII Land with Scott expedition.

1902   Nordenskjold, Otto: South Shetlands, Louis Philippe Land, west Weddell Sea, with Larsen.

       Peary, Robert Edwin: Repulse Bay, Grant Land.

1903   Amundsen, Roald: Canadian Arctic, Beechey Island, Boothia Peninsula, Peel Sound, King William Island ship marooned, overland to Yukon and back to ship, McClintock Strait, Bering Strait, San Francisco, discovered northwest passage to East.

1905   Peary, Robert Edwin: Grant Land, surveyed north Ellesmere Land to Axel Heiberg Island.

Filchner, Wilhelm: Upper Hwang Ho, Szechwan, Shensi, Shansi, Langchow and Kansu.

1907   Shackleton, Ernest Henry: Cape Royds on Ross Island in McMurdo Sound, Mt. Erebus, attempt at the pole via Beardmore Glacier-within 113 miles.

Mawson, Sir Douglas: Ross Barrier, south magnetic pole with Shackleton expedition.

1908   Cook, Frederick: Claimed to be first to reach North Pole, but claim disputed.

Peary, Robert Edwin: Reached North Pole from north tip of Ellesmere Land.

Stefansson, Vilhjalmur: Mackenzie River, Horton River to Coronation Gulf, Victoria Island, Point Barrow.

1910   Scott, Robert Falcon: McMurdo Sound with Wilson, journey to pole via Beardmore Glacier, died in 1912 but expedition continued on.

1911   Amundsen, Roald: Antarctica expedition, Bay of Whales, Ross Barrier, first to reach South Pole.

Mawson, Sir Douglas: Kaiser Wilhelm II Land, Victoria Land in Antarctica, discovered George V and Queen Mary Lands.

1912   Filchner, Wilhelm: Expedition to Weddell Sea, discovered Luitpold Land.

1913   Stefansson, Vilhjalmur: Canadian Arctic expedition, Bering Strait, Beaufort Sea, Prince Patrick Island, discovered an island to north, visited Wrangel Island.

1914   Shackleton, Ernest Henry: Cross Antarctica from Weddell Sea, ship sank, party reached Elephant Island, famous boat voyage to South Georgia.

1918   Amundsen, Roald: Northeast passage to East.

1921   Shackleton, Ernest Henry: Enderby Land, died in South Georgia.

Amundsen, Roald: Attempted to repeat Nansen's drift, to reach North Pole by aircraft, failed.

1925   Amundsen, Roald: Flew with Ellsworth from Spitsbergen over North Pole to Point Barrow.

1926   Byrd, Richard E.: Flight from Spitsbergen to North Pole.

1928   Amundsen, Roald: died while attempting rescue of General Nobile.

1929   Mawson, Sir Douglas: discovered MacRobertson Land.

Byrd, Richard E.: Set up base Little America in Antarctica near Bay of Whales, Marie Byrd Land, Ross Barrier, Queen Maud Range, flight to pole and back.

Fuchs, Sir Vivian: Geologist with Cambridge East Greenland Expedition.

1930   Fuchs, Sir Vivian: East African lakes expedition.

1931   Fuchs, Sir Vivian: East Africa archaeological expedition.

1932   Second International Polar Year

1933   Byrd, Richard E.: Visited Little America.

Fuchs, Sir Vivian: Explored Lake Rudolf in Rift Valley.

1935   Ellsworth, Lincoln: Flew from Dundee Island to Bay of Whales, first man to cross continent by air.

1937   Fuchs, Sir Vivian: Lake Rukwa in East Africa.

1938   Byrd, Richard E.: Surveyed inland from Little America.

1939   Ellsworth, Lincoln: Flights to interior of Antarctica, east of Ross Sea.

1942   Fuchs, Sir Vivian: Went to West Africa.

1947   Byrd, Richard E.: Commanded Operation High Jump.

Fuchs, Sir Vivian: Leader of Falkland Islands Dependencies Survey of Antarctica.

1950   Fuchs, Sir Vivian: Director of Falkland Island Dependencies Survey.

1953   Hillary, Sir Edmund: First to climb Mt. Everest.

1955   Fuchs, Sir Vivian: Leader of Commonwealth Trans-Antarctic Expedition, crossed continent from Weddell Sea to Ross Sea.

1957   Hillary, Sir Edmund: Leader of New Zealand party in Commonwealth Trans-Antarctic Expedition, Scott Base to South Pole.

International Geophysical Year

1961   Antarctic Treaty

summary

Principal Advances in Food and Nutrition

Period	Major Developments in Foods and Nutrition	Major Polar Expeditions
Before 1750	• Sun and oven drying of meats, fruits, and vegetables • Salting of meats and fish, imbedding in fat (pemmican) • Biscuits (hard tack) • Fermentation	• Leif Erikson (circa 1000) • Martin Frobisher (1576–1578) • John Davis (1585–1587) • Willem Barents (1594) • Henry Hudson (1607–1611) • William Baffin (1612–1616) • Vitus Bering (1725–1741)
1750–1815	• Lind experiments recommending lemon juice for treating scurvy • Lemon juice in British Navy rations (1795), but frequently of low ascorbic acid content or limes substituted • Concentrated gelatin (portable soup)	• Samuel Hearne (1770–1772) • Alexander Mackenzie (1789) • James Cook in the South Seas (1772–1775)
1815–1845	• Appert's publication of canning gives canned products for ships—by far the major advancement for expeditions • Bread for ships	• William Perry (1819–1827) • John Ross (1818, 1829–1833) • Fabian von Bellinghausen (1819–1821) • George Back (1833–1837) • James Clark Ross (1839–1843 to Antarctica), (1848–1849) • John Franklin (1819–1827, 1845–1848: all 129 died) • Charles Wilkes (1838–1842 to Antarctica)

Period	Major Developments in Foods and Nutrition	Major Polar Expeditions
1845–1875	• Extensive spoilage of canned British naval stores caused public outcry • Many cans over 10-lb size • Establishment of more rigorous laws and inspections, resulting in only 2–6 lb cans for navy	• John Rae (1846–1854) • Robert McClure (1850–1854) • Elisha Kane (1853–1855) • Leopold McClintock (1857–1859) • Charles Hall (1860–1973) • George Nares (1875–1876) • More than fifty expeditions attempted to solve the mystery of Franklin's disappearance
1875–1900	• Pasteur's findings for microbial spoilage accepted • Better sanitation, inspection and packaging	• George DeLong (1879–1881): a tragedy—two-thirds died from starvation • Adolphus Greely (1881–1884): a tragedy—two-thirds died from starvation • Fridtjof Nansen (1893–1896): crossed Greenland on foot, floated in ship in ice pack across north polar region
1900–1915	• Vitamins recognized, named and accepted by medical profession • Ptomaine theory of cause of scurvy still, however, accepted by a few	• Roald Amundsen (1903–1906): first to make northwest passage and first to South Pole (1911) • Frederick Cook (1907–1909) and Robert Peary (1908–1909) both claimed first to North Pole • Robert Scott (1901–1904) attempt to South Pole: much scurvy; (1910–1913) to South Pole: all five in polar party died of starvation • Ernest Shackleton with Scott in Antarctica in 1901–1904—back in 1907–1909—back in 1914–1916 with open boat voyages to safety • Douglas Mawson (1911–14) in Antarctica—probable hypervitaminosis A from eating dog livers

Period	Major Developments in Foods and Nutrition	Major Polar Expeditions
1915–	• Many vitamins and essential amino acids identified • Extensive general advances in nutrition and food processing, packaging and storage; air travel and refrigeration	• Vihjalmur Stefansson (the "almost Eskimo") (1906–1918): extensive exploration of the Arctic • Richard Byrd (1929–1955) • Opening of Antarctica for international research (1957)

introduction

Food and Exploration

Whether traveling north or south, the polar explorers depended upon their food. Their fate was directly related to the availability and nutritional quality of the food. The best of ships and equipment could not ensure a successful expedition without proper food, and even that was not enough without proper leadership under the frequently harsh and very difficult conditions.

Almost every book on polar exploration contains descriptions of the food. Sometimes emphasis is placed on the food supply, but frequently many writers either did not know or neglected the quality of the food despite its relevance to the success or failure of the whole expedition. Over the centuries of polar exploration, the quality of the food has improved immeasurably, but people still must make decisions about what will be selected and how and when it will be used.

All the advances and changes in food customs as the years went by influenced how well the polar expeditions were supplied. Three major discoveries and their application, however, dramatically changed the health and well-being of polar explorers: the finding (albeit very slowly applied) of Dr. James Lind that lemon juice could cure scurvy, the development of canning by Nicholas Appert, and the discovery by Louis Pasteur that microorganisms caused food to spoil.

Among the more important factors that influenced the decision to explore new lands were the economies of the times, wars, desires for national expansion, national pride, and individual drive for fame and financial reward. From the almost-legendary travels of St. Brendan the Bold in 500 A.D., earlier northern expeditions took place because of the proximity of large populations of technologically advanced people. By the 16th century, sealing was the magnet that attracted hundreds of ships northward.

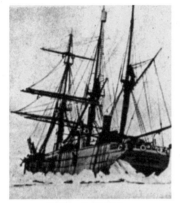

Italian *Stella Polare*

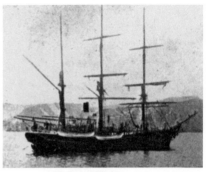

Scottish *Aurora*

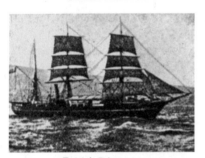

British *Discovery*

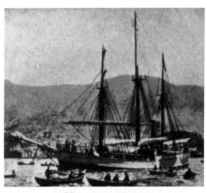

Norwegian *Fram*

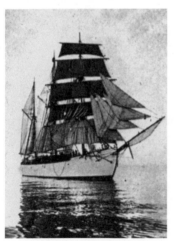

German *Gauss*

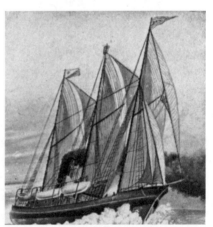

American *Roosevelt*

Comparison of various polar exploring ships.
From R. E. Peary, *Secrets of Polar Travel*, 1917

In the south the magnet was the allure of the South Sea islands and the wealthy trade of the Orient and India.

A plague for most explorers before 1900 was the lack of basic knowledge about nutrition by the medical profession. Common sense, customs, and experience guided those who planned the food. Expedition members learned by trial and error what was good or bad in the foods and materials they encountered. Many were unable to adapt to strange foods or to use the facilities of unknown environments. On long sea travels, and particularly polar expeditions, the choices were often limited. It took many years for information to be interpreted correctly and applied.

Other concerns were food storage and preparation. Food supplies spoiled at high temperatures or were damaged by freezing. Food containers had to be opened and the contents thawed under conditions of low temperatures and high winds. Another difficulty was the preservation of foods for long trips. Decisions had to be made with no knowledge of the stability of vitamins and other important materials in the foods.[1] Nicholas Appert's invention was a crucial turning point in preservation. Some say that the canning industry, together with the addition of lemons in the diet, allowed the British navy to remain at sea for periods long enough to blockade ports successfully and even to win wars.

While science and technology were vital in improving nutrition on polar expeditions, the roles of the administrators and leaders at various levels were also important, in some cases decisive. The British government decided early on to give priority to mastery of the high seas and to exploration. The admiralty in London issued the rules, regulations, and directives for most of England's polar conquests. Politics influenced the opinions, needs, and desires of many. An aging British admiral, for example, would want to send ships back to where he had been to finish some of his work, even though this likely meant failure for the hapless expedition; similar string-pulling often meant failure for other expeditions. The Hudson Bay Company and its board of directors sat in London as well, issuing directives for travel to the Canadian wilderness but with little or no knowledge of the land.[2]

Financing an expedition was also a problem, and some were so poorly financed that there was little to meet the expedition members' needs. Old and worn-out ships were considered good enough to send north into the ice. Purchasing food for expeditions led to difficulties. For the British navy, food purchases had to be let on contract. Price versus quality issues were a constant problem, but the admiralty did a credible job.

Most of the men who led the expeditions did a splendid job. Many were officers from the British navy. Leadership qualities were strained, however, under the stringent conditions of isolation and the constant threat and dire consequences of starvation. Often the best of leaders made serious mistakes, particularly when in areas where their training, expertise, and disposition were not suitable. Careful planning was the key to a successful expedition. According to Robert Peary,

> The detail of equipping a polar expedition is like the detail of equipping an army for foreign service, with, however, this difference. After the expedition has cast loose from civilization there is no chance to rectify mistakes or omissions. No rush wires or cables can be sent back to ship this or that article by next train or steamer. The little ship which bears the hopes of a polar expedition must contain in its restricted space everything to supply all the needs of its people for two or three years in a region where nothing can be obtained but meat, and even that only by those who possess the "know-how." Even when the needs are reduced to almost primeval simplicity, the multiplicity of essential things is great.[3]

Food processing and nutrition have been intertwined forever with armies and navies. Occasionally more time and effort has been spent in supplying food than in fighting. The applications of this knowledge and that of other discoveries during polar explorations were used in ration planning and development for the two world wars of the twentieth century.

Notes

1. Nearly all of what is known about vitamins was discovered after 1900. An entertaining story of the history of vitamin C is described by Kenneth Carpenter in his book *The History of Scurvy and Vitamin C* (Cambridge University Press, 1986).
2. Although mainly covering central and northern Canada, rather than the high polar regions, Peter C. Newman's best seller, *Company of Adventurers* (Penguin Books, 1985), colorfully describes the difficulties caused by this long-range hierarchical administration of affairs.
3. R. E. Peary, *Secrets of Polar Travel* (New York: The Century Company, 1917), 58.

1

The Search for Better Food and Nutrition

An adequate supply of quality food has almost always been the primary need of any group of explorers. Whether they have taken food with them or have had to live off the land, their successes and failures depended on how well they maintained their nutrition. Some would-be experts state that explorers in cold climates have special food requirements. This is not true. The effect of low temperatures is no longer a major problem because modern explorers are dressed in well-insulated clothing that creates a microenvironment similar to what they would have in a warmer climate. Some explorers expend a great amount of physical energy in their explorations, however, and thus need many more calories than usual. These increased calorie requirements, however, are not much greater, or even any greater, than those for people doing very hard work at home.

One of the most serious problems faced by explorers was that of food spoilage. This hampered early expeditions to a great extent and often resulted in starvation and death. Industries did not exist to prepare processed foods. Many fresh foods, such as the obvious ones like meat and vegetables, could not be taken on explorations because they spoiled so quickly. The difficulty caused by food spoilage was interrelated with a nearly complete ignorance of nutrition. Prejudice and greed on the part of those financing and managing the expeditions also contributed to failure.

Early sailors survived the consequences of malnutrition through ingenuity and perseverance. On shorter trips live animals were taken aboard ships for food, but the animals suffered horribly from confinement, inadequate diet, and illness. At least for the officers' messes, some captains had small gardens of vegetables. A diet of fish would sustain many explorers.

Explorers also used dried foods, but the variety was limited, and in many cases their nutritional value was greatly reduced or even destroyed by the drying processes. Properly dried foods were not immune to deteriorative reactions due to the chemistry of the material or the growth of microorganisms.[1]

Where the explorers sought new horizons greatly influenced their provisioning. The requirements differed for those aboard ship versus those traversing land masses. One big difference was, of course, the availability of water. Another was the energy expended to transport the food on land as compared to that expended on a ship. This is probably best shown in the early twentieth century explorations of Captain Robert Falcon Scott and Captain Roald Amundsen, the two who reached the South Pole in 1911–1912. Scott man-hauled his equipment and provisions during the last major part of his trip to and from the pole, while Amundsen used dogs. Many believe the high expenditure of energy and time for man-hauling by Scott's men to have caused their deaths.

The environment also had a very great influence. Obviously one major factor was whether edible materials were available. When comparing the northern and southern polar areas, a principal difference is that the north polar area is a body of water surrounded by land, whereas the south polar area is a body of land surrounded by water. As a result, it is possible for land animals to be far above the Arctic Circle because they can walk across land and even up onto some of the ice during parts of the year, and then they can retreat south, depending upon the season. Seals can also be obtained year-round in the far north. In the south polar region the distance between the land masses to the north and the land mass surrounding the pole is so great that there are no land mammals or reptiles on the antarctic continent. Only sea life ventures upon the shores. As a result of these large differences food can be available part way to and from the North Pole, whereas none is available once the shores of Antarctica are left behind en route to the South Pole.

Early explorers had to contend not only with nutritionally deficient diets aboard ships but even before sailing. Diets for poorer people, the social stratum from which most seamen came, were frequently so inadequate that seamen embarked with nutritional deficiencies.

One of the ways to describe the difference between food and nutrition is by explaining what they are and are not. A person can have an excess of food and yet have poor nutrition, but good nutrition cannot be realized without food. Nutrition is the utilization of foods to supply the body's needs for energy, growth, and good health.

The relationship of the care and preparation of food with the need for adequate nutrition was well recognized in ancient times. Hippocrates, the father of medicine, relates how man had to find the proper foods and ways of processing them in order to survive:

> I hold that the diet and food which people in health now use would not have been discovered, provided it had suited with man to eat and drink in the manner as the ox, the horse, and all other animals, except man, do of the production of the earth, such as fruits, weeds, and grass: for from such things these animals grow, live free of disease, and require no other kind of food. And, at first, I am of the opinion that man used the same sort of food, and that the present articles of diet had been discovered and invented only after a long lapse of time, for when they suffered much and severely from this strong and brutish diet, swallowing things which were raw, unmixed, and possessing great strength, they became exposed to strong pains and diseases, and to early deaths. It is likely, indeed, that from habit they would suffer less from these things then than we would now, but still they would suffer severely even then; and it is likely that the greater number, and those who had weaker constitutions, would all perish; whereas the stronger would hold out for a longer time, as even nowadays some, in consequence of using strong articles of food, get off with little trouble, but others with much pain and suffering. From this necessity it appears to me that they would search out the food befitting their nature, and thus discover that which we now use; and that from wheat, by macerating it, stripping it of its hull, grinding it all down, sifting, toasting, and baking it, they form bread; and from barley they form cake (maza), performing many operations in regard to it; they boiled, they roasted, they mixed, they diluted those things which are strong and of intense qualities with weaker things, fashioning them to the nature and powers of man, and considering that the stronger things Nature would not be able to manage if administered, and that from such things pains, diseases, and death would arise, but such as Nature could manage, that from them food, growth, and health, would arise. To such a discovery and investigation what more suitable name could one give than that of Medicine? Since it was discovered for the health of man, for his nourishment and safety, as the substitute for that kind of diet by which pains, diseases, and deaths were occasioned.[2]

Much of what was considered adequate nutrition before 1700 was learned largely by trial and error. Some physicians made diagnoses that helped to establish what was nutritious, but, by and large, people made their own determination of what was or was not good for them. Serious malnutrition was an obvious consequence of such unenlightened food habits.

Some of the first modern advances in the knowledge of nutrition were made by general practitioners and even by sailors. Scurvy offers a case in point. Long before vitamins were recognized, the occurrence of scurvy was suspected to be related to food. Scurvy, a devastating disease, was known to be the primary (and hideous) threat to sailors on long voyages. Not only disabling but life-threatening, scurvy was dreaded. It was characterized by hemorrhages, especially in the gums and mucous membranes of the mouth accompanied by a spongy condition of the gums, foul breath, loosening of the teeth, stiff joints, swelling of extremities and a general debility, which, if not stopped, concluded in death.

Today scurvy is known to be caused by a deficiency of vitamin C (ascorbic acid), a compound found in plants, especially fruits and leafy vegetables. If previously on a diet adequate in vitamin C, a person can exist as long as ninety days when subjected to a diet highly deficient in the vitamin. As soon as the body's store of vitamin C is depleted, however, symptoms rapidly appear. Although many theories for the cause of the disease had been proposed, only when vitamins in general were recognized in the early 1900s did scientists believe that a nutritional deficiency caused scurvy. It was not until the 1930s that purified ascorbic acid was shown to prevent scurvy.

In spite of this long ignorance of the cause of scurvy, Dr. James Lind, a British surgeon, had reported highly important findings in the 1700s. Dr. Lind is probably the best known of all earlier medical practitioners for work in the field of nutrition. He is considered by many to have conducted the first adequately controlled trial in clinical nutrition, or even in any branch of clinical science, when in 1746 he performed an experiment on twelve sailors with scurvy. All appeared to be afflicted to a similar degree according to his observations.[3] He fed each sailor a similar diet, consisting of gruel with sugar for breakfast; either broth (made with fresh mutton) or pudding for the midday meal; and barley, raisins, rice, currants, and other items in the evening. Two men were allotted to each of six groups for fourteen days. The following were the daily additions to their diets:

Group 1: one quart of alcoholic cider
Group 2: 25 "guts" (about 1 ml) of elixir vitriol, three times during the day
Group 3: two spoonfuls of vinegar three times during the day
Group 4: half a pint of sea water
Group 5: two oranges and one lemon (continued for only 6 days because the supply was exhausted then)
Group 6: a paste (about 4 ml) prescribed by another doctor and consisting of a variety of condiments and flavoring agents, such as garlic and mustard seed; they also drank barley water with additives.[4]

After only six days on the experiment, those receiving oranges and lemons were much improved and were fit for duty, while after fourteen days those receiving cider were healthier than those in the remaining groups. Sailors without any fruit juices did not overcome the symptoms of scurvy.

Lind concluded that oranges and lemons were the most effective scurvy remedies.[5] His observations were not applied until a century and a half later, yet when they were finally used, their validity was questioned and only randomly adopted by the navy, depending upon the captain of the ship. Perhaps Lind's use of only twelve sailors for the experiment was one reason why his work was so poorly accepted.

Even Lind himself did not see that scurvy was caused by a nutritional deficiency but rather thought that it was a disease that oranges and lemons could cure. Many of the erroneous theories for scurvy's cause existed for another century and a half, including what has been called the group of pneumatic theories concerning the effect of gases. Perhaps the earliest of the pneumatic theories was that carbonated water cured scurvy. Nonmedical scientists became involved in the scurvy debates, and when Joseph Priestley, a well-accepted English scientist of the time, found that he could make soda water by shaking it with "fixed air" (carbon dioxide), then a lack of oxygen in tissues was claimed to be responsible for the symptoms of scurvy. Oxygen-containing acids were soon substituted for fixed air, and carbonated water was used aboard ships.

The utilization of lemon juice as a successful remedy for scurvy was then thought by some to be due to its content of organic acids containing oxygen. In one reported experiment, scurvy was treated successfully when citric acid (a high-oxygen-containing acid) was dissolved in lemon juice. The lemon juice, of course, was thought merely to be the supplier of more citric acid.

Still other theories included one claiming that eating putrefied food caused scurvy.[6] Yet another hypothesis, but one with little support, was that metal poisoning caused scurvy due to contamination with copper. This was the result of observations that when foods were cooked in copper kettles, scurvy was more rampant. This observation is now known to be true—but for different reasons. Even until the early 1900s, preparations of lemon juice were exposed to copper piping and stored in air, conditions now known to destroy vitamin C.

In 1768, Captain James Cook led a scientific expedition to the South Pacific to test the value of a variety of suspected antiscorbutics—remedies against scurvy—including sauerkraut, portable soup (meat extract dried in slabs like a glue), malt, oranges, and lemons.[7] His expedition was a large one and not a single man died of scurvy, but he fed his men a variety of fresh fruit as the ships went from island to island. As a result of his very successful trip, lemons and oranges on board ship were not considered necessary to prevent scurvy, even by Cook. He, therefore, took along with him Priestley's equipment for making soda water as an antiscorbutic.

It took many years before Lind's experiments were put to practical use. Food science and technology had not yet progressed to the point that lemon and orange juices could be processed effectively to ensure the presence of adequate amounts of vitamin C.

It was not until 1882 when another physician, Kanehiro Takaki of the Japanese navy, showed that the disease beriberi—caused by a B-vitamin (thiamine) deficiency—could be cured by eating more vegetables, fish, meat, and unpolished rice. In 1890, a Dutch researcher, Christaan Eijkman, in Java showed that chickens fed polished rice became ill, but when fed unpolished rice they did not. The symptoms of the illness that he called polyneuritis were loss of balance and paralysis. Most important, Eijkman showed that he could cure the disease by feeding the chickens a combination of polished rice together with the polishings. This was the first experiment showing that a particular part of a food item was important. Since then many of the vitamins now known to be the important constituents in those fractions of foods that are essential have been discovered, and the procedures for discovering them refined.

Today at least nine water-soluble vitamins, four fat-soluble vitamins, and over sixteen mineral elements have been identified. These microsubstances are essential to health and well being. Also essential are the macrosubstances: carbohydrates, proteins and fats, plus that very important substance, water. Energy, derived mainly from fat and carbohydrates, and catalysts like vitamins, are necessary. Building blocks, like proteins and some minerals like calcium and phosphate, are also necessary. The vitamins, with the exception of ascorbic acid, are required in very small amounts (the human body cannot synthesize large quantities) and they generally serve as helpers or parts of catalysts, rather than as substances used for energy or structural developments. Some mineral elements also function this way.

Proteins consist of amino acids that have many different structures, and different proteins do not contain the same mixture of amino acids. Since certain amino acids are like certain vitamins in that the human body cannot synthesize them, some proteins are much more nutritious than others. But

Table 1.1
Classification of nutrients. From Wenck et al (1980)

	MACRO-NUTRIENTS	
	Nutrients	
	Carbohydrates (sugar and starch; also fiber)	
	Proteins	
	Fats	
	Water	
MICRO-NUTRIENTS	**Water** Soluble	**Fat** Soluble
Vitamins	Vitamin C (ascorbic acid)	A
	Niacin	D
	Thiamin	E
	Riboflavin	K
	Folic acid (or	
	Folacin)	
	Pantothenic acid	
	Pyridoxine (B_6)	
	B_{12}	
	Biotin	
ELEMENTS	MACRO-ELEMENTS	MICRO-ELEMENTS
Mineral Elements	Calcium	Iron
	Phosphorus	Manganese
	Sodium	Copper
	Potassium	Iodine
	Chlorine	Fluorine
	Sulfur	Zinc
	Magnesium	Cobalt
		Molybdenum
		Selenium

at the time of the polar explorers, these differences in the amino acid contents of proteins were not known.[8]

On strenuous polar expeditions, sufficient food energy was a serious nutritional difficulty for many explorers. High-calorie foods from fat and carbohydrates supplied this energy, but they had to be easy to carry and to prepare under very cold and difficult conditions. An explorer's diet would not qualify as balanced by today's standards. It is recognized today that deficiencies in a single nutrient can affect the requirements for other nutrients. Many other relationships must also be considered, such as how some substances can make other substances physiologically unavailable. For example, calcium can be strongly affected by oxalic acid found in some leafy vegetables like spinach.

Nutritional inadequacy and insufficient food energy were only two of the causes of the nutritional problems experienced by early explorers. Excess vitamin A was another hazard for polar explorers; a pathology named hypervitaminosis A quickly appeared in men who ate the livers of some animals whose diet originated from marine creatures.

Diseases interplayed with nutritionally caused pathologies. Under the stress of poor assimilation of foods because of diarrhea, nutritional deficiencies were exacerbated. Under the stress of nutritional deficiency, infections (such as those causing diarrhea) could have been increased, and so on. Though infections were encountered especially in the early ships in the tropics, they afflicted northern voyagers as well.

Because vitamins were unknown, and indeed, the whole concept of essential catalysts was not recognized during the times of explorations before the early 1900s, the reasons why these explorers suffered serious nutritional deficiencies are clear. Studies to determine the nutritional needs of people generally, as well as those exposed to extreme environments and with high energy needs, continue today. For more information, see appendix A and B.

Notes

1. People of the last half of the 20th century are so accustomed to the many advances in food technology in manufacturing processed foods that it is difficult for them to comprehend fully what was not available years ago. Modern food technology not only processes many varieties of foodstuffs but it does so in a way that retains most of their nutritional qualities as well as their physical and functional properties. These properties are frequently not appreciated, but they are equally as important because people will not eat what they do not enjoy unless they are starving. Foods must be restored to their original form as much as possible, even giving the impression that

they are fresh. This includes the entire process of mastication, how the food feels when it is chewed and how the saliva wets the food. Functional properties include those that are important in cooking, such as forming gels or foams through beating or whipping.

2. "Hippocrates," in *On Ancient Writings*, Section 3, Circa 390 B.C. Translated by Francis Adams in *The Great Books* (Chicago: University of Chicago and Encyclopedia Britannica Inc., 1982), 10.

3. K. J. Carpenter, *The History of Vitamin C* (Cambridge University Press, 1986), 52.

4. Ibid.

5. Ibid., 53.

6. The putrefaction theory was held by some even until the time of Captain Robert Scott, in the early twentieth century.

7. J. C. Beaglehole, *The Life of Captain James Cook* (Stanford: Stanford University Press, 1974), 135.

8. K. J. Carpenter, *Protein and Energy* (Cambridge: Cambridge University Press, 1994), 124.

2

Food Processing, Preservation, and Polar Exploration

The preparation and preservation of foods are among the oldest arts. Near the Great Pyramids of Cheops in Egypt is a tomb with walls engraved with depictions of foods of the time.[1] Scenes depict grinding flour, baking bread, brewing beer, and killing and cooking cattle and poultry. Not only did people in ancient times practice such arts, they also knew something about food preservation. They had to. Food was preserved to provide an uninterrupted supply in winter or during other periods of unavailability. Of all the methods that were used, drying was one of the easiest and most successful. Not only did it frequently provide foods with at least moderate stability during storage, but it also provided foods that were deydrated and thus easily transported over long distances. This led to their use by nomadic tribes and by explorers of the time.

Although fruits were relatively more expensive and their keeping qualities were not high, they were included aboard earlier ships. Dried fruits are described in many of the stories from the older Arabian countries and from Asia. Dried figs, raisins, and apricots are discussed in stories from Mesopotamia in central Asia. Most of these were dried in the sun, a procedure that went well with the seasons and places where they grew, which provided hot sun and dry air.

Fish and some meats were preserved through drying. A variation was drying that included smoking. One of the earliest ways of treating fish was to salt them, sometimes together with drying. The famous stockfish, used aboard many ships even up to the middle 1800s, were prepared in this manner. Dairy products are also a relatively old commodity; people learned early how to make cheeses. Other aged products have been available since the beginning of history. Ancient Egyptians had a type of beer, and the presence of wine is noted throughout historical and religious writings. Here

15

the alcohol content offered some degree of preservation. Probably one of the best fermented products for sailors was sauerkraut, a product of a lactic-acid bacterial fermentation. Sauerkraut has at least a moderate level of vitamin C, and the mildly acidic conditions offer a preservative medium for this vitamin.[2]

The North American Indians are credited with developing a simple meat product called pemmican. This early means of preserving meats was literally to embed them in fat.[3] This sometimes required melting the fat and mixing it thoroughly with lean meat. As much as fifty to sixty percent of the product could be fat. The value of embedding the meat in fat was probably in the exclusion of oxygen. The type of fat used was important in order to cut down the oxidative effects. Although not the same as the Indian product, high-fat meat preparations were also found in other parts of the world.

It has been reported that the original pemmican was invented by the Cree and was made of the dried meat of buffalo, caribou, and deer. Later, after the buffalo had been largely exterminated by the white man, beef was used. The meat was first dried in the sun and then pounded and cut up before being mixed with melted fat.

Pemmican saved the lives of many North American explorers. It was an important food product because it was compact and high in energy. For long storage and easy carrying on a person's back, pemmican was tightly packed in eighty-pound sacks made of buffalo hide. Dried fruits were often added to improve preservation; the Indians incorporated dried acid berries. Later on, when pemmican was made in England and packaged for use aboard ship by British explorers, other types of fruits and condiments were added. The Eskimos used a similar product made of small pieces of seal meat.

In the early days, pemmican was such a highly valued food that it was even used in trade as a medium of financial exchange.[4] The white men bought it from the Indians, then traded it among themselves and even back to the Indians. To the Indians, pemmican was a miracle food. They saved it for eating on ceremonial occasions or used it as an emergency food to avert famine. Explorers, trappers, and fur traders relished it on their trips. Apparently they became accustomed to the taste and benefitted from the high-calorie content. It was so valuable that control of its supply even caused what has been described as the "First Pemmican War." The conflict was between two rival trading outfits, the Hudson Bay Company and the Northwest Company, during the early 1800s. Only in 1821 when the two companies joined to establish the enlarged Hudson Bay Company did peace arrive. In North Dakota, where the selling of pemmican was paramount, a town was even named after it—Pembina.

In some form or another, most of the preserved meats were used by early explorers. Unfortunately, the drying procedures sometimes caused extensive loss of nutritive value. On land, early explorers knew that they should also sample and eat grains and berries along their routes. Sometimes they even got fresh meat.

In 1804, the following weekly provision allowance was recommended by the British Navy for each man:

Food Item	Quantity/Week
Brisket, salt	7 pounds
Beer	7 gallons, wine measure
Beef, salt	4 pounds
Pork, salt	2 pounds
Peas	2 pints
Oatmeal	3 pints
Butter	6 ounces
Cheese	12 ounces
Vinegar	1/2 pint

This gave 4,500 kilocalories per day, but the calculations are uncertain, and in at least one case and probably many more, the butter and cheese were replaced with tea, sugar, and cocoa, greatly lowering the nutritional value of the diet, which was at best nutritionally a very poor one.[5]

Since fruits have a high acidity, which retards the growth of the more dangerous bacteria, it was much easier to preserve them than it was to preserve foods like meats. Bottling of fruits was done very early. In ancient times fruits were preserved in honey or another sugar-containing material, with very little heating. A big problem was how to seal the bottles, but shortly after 1700 there were many extensively used home procedures for bottling different fruits.

Sometime around 1750 the Dutch navy started using foods packed in iron containers. The procedure for packaging was to cook the material and, while it was hot, to put it in a can and cover it with hot fat. Then the lid was soldered on. This was later extended to preserving salmon in a similar way.

Shortly after 1800, Thomas Saddington in London was awarded a prize for an inexpensive procedure for preserving fruit without sugar. This procedure was available for home use as well as sea stores. The procedure used methods which involved careful control of heating and sealing of the containers. It is possible that Saddington's procedure would have been widely adopted if not for the extensive work of Nicholas Appert. Saddington's process was a financial success nonetheless.

A turning point occurred in the early 1800s when canning was developed by Nicholas Appert, which increased the variety, availability, and quality of preserved foods. Before then, preserved foods were costly and were used mainly by the very rich or in naval or other expeditions. His discovery was received with great enthusiasm by French naval circles just after 1800. Appert, a Frenchman, had spent seven years developing his procedure before submitting his trials to the navy minister in Paris. Unfortunately those results were initially expected to be used only for sick sailors, not for general distribution. In his book, *The Art of Preserving* (1812) he describes the stages of the process.

1. Enclos[e] in bottles the substance to be preserved.

2. [Cork] the bottles with the utmost care, for it is chiefly on the corking that the success of the process depends.

3. [Submit] these enclosed substances to the action of boiling water in water bath (baliem marie) for a greater or less length of time, according to their nature, and in the manner pointed out with respect to each several kind of substance.

4. [Withdraw] the bottle from the water bath at the time described.[6]

He also described his home laboratory and production plant, with recommendations on how to adapt the canning procedure for home use. He had a special section on "bottles and vessels," preferring glass "as being the matter most impenetrable by air...."

The ordinary bottles have generally necks too small and ill-made; they are also too weak to resist the blows from the bat [used to pound the corks in] and the action of the fire. I, therefore, caused bottles to be made for my especial use with wider necks, and those necks with a projecting rim or ring on the interior surface placed below and resembling, in form, the rim which is at the top of the exterior surface of the necks of bottles. My object was that when the cork had been forced into the neck of the bottle three-fourths of its length in the manner already described it should be compressed in the middle.[7]

He goes on to give more information on the bottles as well as the corks, emphasizing how important it was to close the bottles properly. His products were submitted to a variety of tests by the French Maritime Prefect.[8]

When canneries opened in Britain, they started using not only glass bottles but tin and iron cannisters as well.[9] At least initially, cans were adopted to utilize the iron of English factories, not because they were sturdier and would withstand freezing better than glass on polar expeditions. The iron cannisters, or tin cans as they became known (even though the early ones were heavy iron), were a major advance. In the canning procedure the lid of the can was initially left with a vent hole. The can was heated in boiling water for a prolonged period, up to six hours, with its vent hole above the water level. When no more air came out, the top of the can was then soldered closed. Not only was solder used to seal the airhole left at the top of the can but also to seal the seams of the cans, all of this by hand.[10] Initial reports on the use of the canned products were enthusiastic. Since solder contains lead, however, one wonders how much lead ended up in the contents of a particular can. One instance where lead probably got into canned food was a report on the possible lead poisoning of the crew of the *Jeannette* in the Arctic from eating canned tomatoes.[11] The tomatoes were found to contain small pieces of solder, supposedly loosened by the acid of the tomato. In another report by Sir Joseph Banks to the Duncan Hall and Gambal Company, the findings are less ominous:

> The cannister of roasted filet of veal you sent me on January 15, 1813, appeared to have been put up on December 5, 1812, and after remaining in my possession for two years and six months was yesterday opened and declared by the unanimous voice of the party present to be in perfect state of preservation and had not lost any of its nutritious qualities.[12]

Foods were packaged in enormous cans soon thereafter. In 1850 Captain Robertson of the East India Company's ship *Surat Castle* received one can weighing 13 lbs. 14 ozs., another one 17 lbs. 8 ozs., another 16 lbs., and so forth. The large sizes of these cans led to the problem of inadequate sterilization.[13]

The most important early data on canned foods came from their use by the merchant marine, and later from some problems with long-term storage. It was in Parry's expedition to the Northwest Passage in 1818 that the first real test occurred.[14] Parry gave a positive report on the canned foods, and in later trips he also had the same result, giving strong support for their value.

Then there was the famous southern trip by James Ross in 1839. Ross had twenty-six tons of canned food. He had a problem with some of the cans being too thin, but he still found them better than the former naval supplies.[15]

One of the great chemists of the time, Louis Gay Lussac, probably set back advances by suggesting that it was only the presence of oxygen that caused putrefaction in cans, and he believed that heating cans in boiling water drove out the oxygen.

> Animal and vegetable materials shown contact with air promptly begin to putrefy and ferment. By exposing them to the temperature of boiling in hermetically sealed vessels, the absorbed oxygen produces a new combination which is no longer likely to produce fermentation or putrefaction when it becomes fixed by heat in a similar way to albumin.[16]

If air could be removed from large cans, he thought, everything would be all right. It is now known that merely removing the air might not ensure heating of the contents adequate to kill the microorganisms responsible for spoilage.

By the 1840s the problem of spoilage was recognized. Supplies used on naval assignments often spoiled because the cans were too large for proper sterilization. Even today cans of fifteen to twenty-five pound capacity are very difficult to sterilize. It also was not known at the time that the temperature of the food was an important aspect of the canning process.[17] Sanitation problems resulted from microbial contamination as well, plus the presence of undesirable materials such as entrails, hair, feet, and claws.

Awareness of these problems led to the conclusion that the Franklin expedition, which was then lost in the Arctic, could have died from food poisoning. It was later shown that the members of the expedition obtained many of their supplies from one company in central Europe. The canned goods were produced in Moldavia, not in England. There was evidence, however, that two kinds of canned goods were made, one of high quality for the navy and another for the general public that was made more cheaply, possibly with less heating. Soon the navy established its own inspection groups, and cans of only seven or eight pound capacity were purchased. Slowly Australian canned meat products became available in England and the rest of Europe; rather than waste the remains of cattle slaughtered only for their hides, the meat was preserved in cans. Canned foods were now a world-wide, fairly safe, and generally available commodity.

The work of Gail Borden and Louis Pasteur revolutionized food processing by supplying safer and less perishable food. Gail Borden introduced the canning of condensed milk. Pasteur's work resulted in the finding that putrefaction came from spores and materials in the air; the process he developed for the treatment of milk by heat bears his name, pasteurization.

Following this, it was possible to begin examining food products, even with the crude microbiological methods of the day, to assess the adequacy of sterilization. Pasteur's contributions also helped to formulate procedures for processing foods that destroy micoorganisms that cause food-borne disease.

Both scientists' work aided in the development of a particular food product, processed milk. As with canned meats and milk, pasteurized milk could be safely distributed to the rapidly increasing population of urban areas. From 1800 to 1900 there were very large increases, usually about tenfold, in the populations of European towns, particularly in England. This resulted in a large increase in the food requirements for these growing urban populations, which in turn resulted in a greater economic need to preserve foods long enough for these populations to use them. Even so, the urban poor suffered greatly from malnutrition throughout the entire 19th century. It was not until the beginning of the 20th century that the nutrition of these people improved, mainly because of technical advances.

Notes

1. J. H. Breasted, "The rise of man," *Science* 74 (1931): 639–43. See also G. Lusk, *Nutrition* (New York: Paul B. Hueber, 1933).
2. Sauerkraut was supplied on Captain Cook's famous voyage to the South Pacific in the 1700s. Perhaps this is one of the reasons why the crew members maintained good health, which contributed to the success of the voyage.
3. For additional information, see V. Fisher, *Pemmican* (Garden City, N.Y.: Doubleday and Co., 1956); and E. F. Binkerd, O.E. Kolari, and C. Tracy, "Pemmican," *Maricopa Trails* 1, 1 (1977): 1–10.
4. Binkerd, Kolari, and Tracy, 6. Some did not share the early explorers' enthusiasm for this product. Vilhjalmur Stefansson was met with strong rebuffs when he ardently promoted pemmican for the U.S. military at the beginning of World War II; modern food technology could not accept such an ancient product. In several tests, products called pemmican were found unpleasant by volunteer test groups. It was better accepted, however, when eaten during difficult and treacherous journeys.
5. S. Thorne, *The History of Food Preservation* (Cumbria, England: Parthenon Publication Group Ltd., 1986).
6. M. Appert, *The Art of Preserving*, Report of the Board of Arts and Manufacture, Paris. Translated from the French (London: Black, Parry and Kingsbury, 1812).
7. Ibid., 18.
8. Ibid.
9. J. C. Drummond and W. E. Lewis, "The examination of some tinned foods of historic interest, part I," *Chemistry and Industry* (August 27, 1938): 808–15.
10. O. Beattie and J. Geiger, *Frozen in Time* (Saskatoon, Canada: Western Producer Prairie Books, 1987), 173.

11. L. F. Guttridge, *Icebound. The Jeannette Expedition's Quest for the North Pole* (Annapolis: Naval Institute Press, 1986), 173.

12. S. Thorne, *The History of Food Preservation*, 40.

13. J. C. Drummond and W. E. Lewis, 809.

14. W. E. Parry, *Three Voyages for the Discovery of the Northwest Passage ...in 1819–20* (New York: Harper & Brothers, 1821), 402.

15. S. Thorne, 52.

16. In one case, upon opening 643 cans, 573 were condemned and examination of more of these revealed that frequently over 90 percent were unsafe.

17. S. Thorne, 58.

3

Early Exploration

Since the earliest times, exploration has been driven by a desire to learn what is beyond one's horizons and to experience the thrill of the search for the unknown. The dangers of early exploration included not only confrontations with wild animals, shipwrecks, and drownings but also serious food problems.

Although many of the conditions encountered in polar explorations were very different from those encountered in warmer climates, the experiences of explorers in the latter were still useful to their poleward-trekking colleagues. Early expeditions were usually a combination of a search for new lands in which to live and/or hunt for treasure. Sea voyages were common in the Mediterranean Sea several thousand years ago. In 1600 B.C., the Phoenicians were probably the first to sail around Africa. They supplemented their food supply by stopping in distant locations at proper intervals to raise crops.[1]

Not much is recorded on seafaring activities in the Atlantic until the legend of the Irish monk, St. Brendan of Clonfert, in the 6th century.[2] Unfortunately, a written account of Brendan's sea voyages does not exist, though his wanderings are firmly entrenched in Ireland's mythic history. Many believe that Brendan's voyages are not just legend because there is evidence of an Irish explorer who lived before the Vikings, and Brendan actually lived in southwest Ireland in about 500 A.D. Celtic monks at that time strove to be martyrs and sometimes lived as hermits. To achieve martyrdom, they set themselves adrift in boats with the belief that God would lead them to a proper divine future. According to legend, Brendan set himself adrift around 550 A.D. with fourteen other monks. At the time, he was about sixty years old.[3]

The monks were probably as hard boiled as any seaman anyone has ever known and were dedicated ascetics. Brendan may have had several voyages, but one he is known to have taken was around the Shetland and the Faeroe Islands. According to the accounts, he and the monks who accompanied him left the islands then continued west for forty days, probably arriving off the coast of Newfoundland, where they saw icebergs. Then they traveled south by Nova Scotia and reported strange animals, probably walruses. Continuing further south along the coast, perhaps even to Florida, they reported wild vines heavy to the ground with grapes. The monks' diet while at sea is not known, but they probably carried some dried fruits and periodically were able to fish. Along the coast of America, supplies from their ventures on shore were bountiful. Other stories of Irish monks traveling on the northern shores of America are known, possibly to escape the advancing Vikings, who reported that they found evidence of habitation in the Americas.

The Viking discovery of the northern section of the North American continent is still a cloudy mix of some recognized artifacts and multicolored tales from Norse sagas. The location of the famous Leif Ericson's Vineland has been claimed to be in many places over a thousand-mile range of coastland.

The Vikings were known earlier as a dreaded scourge in Europe when they sailed their longships along the British and European coasts, and even into the Mediterranean Sea. These longships, however, were not the ones used by the Viking explorers of the New World. These were instead a vessel called the knorr which were as much as 100 feet long and capable of carrying forty tons of cargo. As many as sixty oarsmen, as well as a square sail, navigated them through the worst of adverse weather.[4]

Some say as many as 40,000 Vikings lived in Iceland around 1000 A.D. They were also in Greenland as much as 100 years earlier. One of the most well known, Eric the Red (Eric Thorvaldsson), is credited with naming the island Greenland in 982 on a visit with not only a crew but livestock to provide fresh meat for the trip. He traveled to Greenland from Iceland to distance himself from a conflict with his farming neighbors. His flotilla included twenty-five ships carrying as many as 700 men, women, and children and a large stock of cattle, goats, chickens, and horses. Only half of the ships arrived safely. The Norse disappearance from Greenland in the 15th century may be due to the isolation in small groups, though problems associated with the food and harsh climate must have contributed to their demise as well.[5]

Another Viking explorer, Leif Ericson, the son of Eric the Red and a sturdy "dreamlander" (a natural explorer, always pursuing faraway places), is usually credited with naming the part of the Labrador coast known as Markland (meaning Woodland), and then Vineland further down the American coast. A great controversy exists over the true location of Vineland. Wherever it was, apparently there was little or no snow in winter, and when Ericson left he carried a load of timber and what he called dried grapes.[6]

A period followed where many of the explorations took place on land in Europe, Africa, and the Orient. In the 15th century, however, Portugal became a seafaring center, and the Portuguese began to send their ships into the more distant Atlantic. Christopher Columbus learned to sail while at his native town, Genoa in Italy, but later moved to Portugal. He had to turn to Spain, however, for financing his visits to the Americas. Queen Isabella of Spain supported his well-known expedition with three caravels in 1492. Events then moved quickly, and by the time of Columbus' fourth voyage in 1503, the English were on the northern shore of America. Financed by Bristol merchants, John Cabot and his son, Sebastian, were regular visitors to the Americas.

Sea expeditions now proceeded in many southern waters. To further Portugal's claim to fame and power, Vasco da Gama set out to sail around Africa in 1497. His fleet had 180 men in four ships, each over 100 tons. The voyage took more than 300 days on the open sea and covered nearly 25,000 miles. This voyage produced the first extensive report of bad cases of scurvy, which were undoubtedly related to the crews' being at sea for nearly 100 days in one stretch.[7] Three months without fresh foods or supplements high in vitamin C was enough time for the onset of serious symptoms of scurvy.

Portugal, a nation of fishermen, again refused to support an individual who later became one of the most famous seamen and explorers, Ferdinand Magellan. The king of Spain finally supported Magellan's plan to sail around the world. In 1519 he sailed in five ships, each of about 100 tons displacement, with a crew of 280 men, mostly Spaniards. After one ship was wrecked and another one deserted, Magellan finally found an outlet from the South Atlantic into the Pacific Ocean the following spring. Moving up along the west coast of South America and out into the open Pacific, they sailed for ninety-six days before reaching the Ladrone Islands north of the equator—

three months without a landfall and fresh food. An Italian named Pigafetta wrote in his diary:

> Wednesday, November 28, 1520, we debouched from that strait, engulfing ourselves in the Pacific Sea. We were three months and twenty days without getting any kind of fresh food. We ate biscuit, which was no longer biscuit, but powder of biscuits swarming with worms, for they had eaten the good. It stank strongly of the urine of rats. We drank yellow water that had been putrid for many days. We also ate some ox hides that covered the top of the mainyard to prevent the yard from chafing the shrouds, and which had become exceedingly hard because of the sun, rain, and wind. We left them in the sea for four or five days, and then placed them for a few moments on top of the embers, and so ate them; and often we ate sawdust from boards. Rats were sold for one-half ducado apiece, and even then we could not get them. But above all the other misfortunes the following was the worst. The gums of both the lower and upper teeth of some of our men swelled, so that they could not eat under any circumstances and therefore died. Nineteen men died from that sickness. Twenty-five or thirty men fell sick in the arms, legs, or in another place, so that but a few remained well. However, I, by the grace of God, suffered no sickness. We sailed about four thousand leagues during those three months and twenty days through an open stretch in that Pacific Sea.[8]

Pigafetta's diary entry describes extreme cases of scurvy. Possibly the rats saved a few lives, for rats are very high in vitamin C. Less than two weeks later the survivors landed in the Philippines. Unfortunately, Magellan was killed by natives on a small island, and the situation deteriorated in the commander's absence. Later, when the one remaining ship reached home, Magellan was nearly forgotten. His exploits were recognized only much later in history.

Explorations became diversions from the tracks of previous voyages along the coast of Africa and the Americas. A possible shortcut to the fabulous Orient over the top of North America became one major objective. This, in turn, required more extensive expeditions into hazardous areas and offered serious problems with survival.

Notes
  1. Herodotus, circa 450 B.C., *The History*, in *Of Herodotus, Great Books of the Western World*, R. M. Hutchins, ed. (Chicago: Encyclopedia Britannica, Inc., 1982), 131.
  2. Benedeit, *The Anglo-Norman Voyage of St. Brendan*, I. Short and B. Merrilees, ed. (Manchester: Manchester University Press, 1979), 4.
  3. Ibid., 5.
  4. L. F. Hannon, *The Discoverers* (Toronto: McClelland and Stewart, Ltd., 1971), 36.

5. F. Hødnebø and J. Kristjánsson, ed., *The Vikings Discovery of America* (Oslo: J. M. Stenersens Forlag A/S, 1991), 278, 280.

6. A written description of the Vikings' travels was not made until several hundred years after their voyages. At least in the northern tip of Newfoundland, archaeological work has provided proof of a settlement.

7. F. Debenheim, *Discovery and Exploration* (London: Geographical Projects, Ltd., 1960), 66.

8. A. Pigafetta, *Magellan's Voyage Around the World* (Cleveland: The Arthur H. Clark Company, 1906), 83–84.

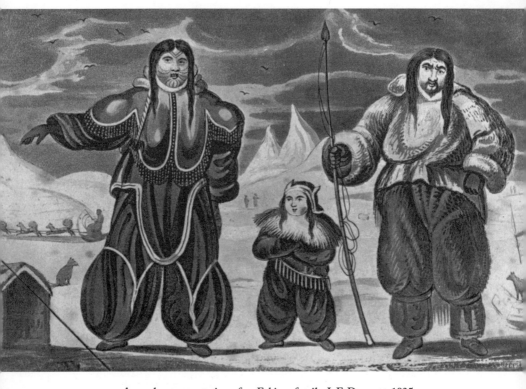

An early representation of an Eskimo family. J. F. Dennett, 1835.

4

The Eskimos

Historically, the peoples of the far north have been masters of adaptation.[1] They survived under conditions that included not only cold temperatures and icy, barren terrain, but for some, seasonal periods of complete darkness. Survival depended upon adequate clothing and shelter for protection against extreme conditions and upon the availability of food.

The early whalers and explorers did not understand the customs of these northern people nor their ability to clothe, feed, and protect themselves. In *Arctic Dreams: Imagination and Desire in an Arctic Landscape*, Barry Lopez describes their beliefs:

> The sophistication the whalers felt next to the Eskimo was a false sophistication, and presumptuous. The European didn't value the Eskimo's grasp of the world. And, however clever Eskimos might be with ivory implements and waterproof garments, he thought their techniques dated or simply quaint next to his own. A ship's officer of the time wrote summarily that the Eskimo was 'dwindled in his form, his intellect, and his passions.' They were people to be taken mild but harmless advantage of, to be chastised like children, but not to be taken seriously. The Europeans called them yaks.
>
> As for the Eskimo, they thought the whalers strange for trying to get on without the skills and companionship of women. They gave them full credit for producing 'valuable and convenient articles and implements,' but laughed at their inability to clothe, feed, and protect themselves. They regarded the whalers with a mixture of *ilira* and *kappia*, the same emotions a visitor to the modern village of Pond Inlet encounters today. *Ilira* is the fear that accompanies awe; *kappia* is fear in the face of unpredictable violence. Watching a polar bear—*ilira*. Having to cross thin sea ice—*kappia*.[2]

Those whalers and explorers who had the good sense to do so, however, adopted many of the Eskimos' ways of living.[3]

Just as each group of Eskimos had distinctive customs, the diet of each group was determined by the environment. E. M. Weyer describes a

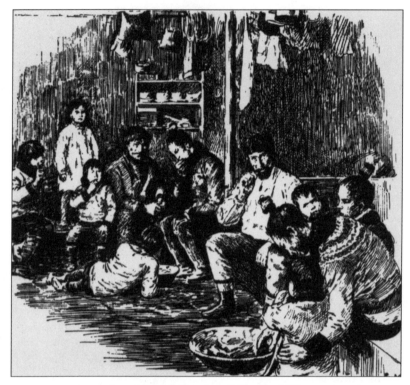

A meal in an Eskimo hut. F. Nansen, 1892

variety of common foodstuffs in his book, *The Eskimos, Their Environment and Folkways*:

> They derive their sustenance from all the natural world of their environment: they hunt mammals, both of the land and sea, obtain fish from fresh and salt water, and supplement these activities by securing birds and their eggs. In certain districts they even draw upon the scanty plant foods of their habitat, gathering berries and collecting roots and herbs. All these sources combined supply food enough for only a very sparse population. The Eskimos did well at the Arctic frontier of the habitable world.[4]

With the exception of some groups, such as those who lived on favored locations along the coast, the food supply did not allow many Eskimos to remain in one place, and they migrated long distances to find their quarry. The seasons determined where they searched for food.

A common factor among all groups was that they ate their foods fresh and often raw.[5] According to *Webster's Third New International Dictionary*, the word Eskimo means, roughly, "eaters of raw flesh."[6] Eating meat raw was sometimes necessary when materials to cook it were not readily available. In some cases, raw meat simply was preferred. Even though the practice was not widespread, the Eskimos' consumption of raw meat may have protected them from deteriorative changes in the food from cooking, such as losses in vitamins, or the formation of carcinogens from cooking over an open fire.

Vilhjalmur Stefansson was not an unprejudiced supporter of eating raw meat. He wrote that "admittedly the whole diet of a strictly carnivorous group of Eskimos provided more raw or rare meat than ours contains, but we eat many raw or hardly cooked items also. We eat soft-boiled eggs, while the Eskimos cook theirs hard. Our roasts are rarer than theirs. They ate much raw, but when it was convenient, the Eskimos cooked."[7] Stefansson observed that some groups of Eskimos added plants to their diet when meat was scarce or unavailable. A dish made from the contents of a caribou's stomach (twigs, grass, moss, and suchlike), immersed in oil and allowed to ferment, was considered a delicacy; it resembled soft Camembert.[8] Undercooked meat or the salad-like acidic mixture of grasses and plants were scurvy palliatives.

In Greenland, the Inuit diet was based mainly on food from the ocean. Nansen described this in some detail:

> One feature of the Greenlanders' daily life, which to us seems strange enough, is that they have no fixed meal times; they simply eat when they are hungry if there is anything to be had. They have a remarkable power of doing without food, but to make up for this they can consume at a sitting astonishing quantities of meat, blubber, fish, and so forth. Their cookery is simple and easy to learn. Meat and fish are sometimes eaten raw or frozen, sometimes boiled and sometimes dried; sometimes meat is allowed to undergo a sort of decomposition or fermentation, when it is called *mikiak*, and is eaten without further preparation. Addition of this sort, which is very highly esteemed, is rotten seal heads. The blubber of seals and whales is generally eaten raw. Of vegetable food, the primitive Greenlanders used several sorts; in addition to angelica, I may mention dandelions, sorrel, crowberries, bilberries, and different kinds of seaweeds. One of their greatest delicacies is the contents of a reindeer's stomach.[9]

Not only did Eskimos eat their food fresh, they also preserved it by freezing or drying. Weyer observes that these and a variety of other methods were used successfully.

> Cached provisions represent a sort of insurance by smoothing out the season inequalities in the productivity of hunting. At Point Barrow meat is

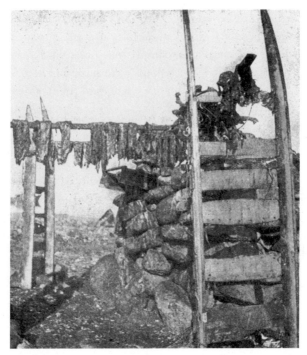

Eskimo at Etah drying meat out of reach of dogs and polar bears. C. Morris, 1909.

stored in great subterranean digs so deep that it remains frozen throughout the summer. The Copper Eskimos commonly cache their stores on top of rock piles so that wild animals cannot plunder them. In Labrador reindeer meat is dried in the spring and frozen in the autumn.[10]

Survival was enhanced through cooperation among groups and a willingness to share provisions in times of need.

(1) hunting grounds, or rather the privilege of hunting on them, is a communal right except in rather rare instances; (2) the hunters almost always have the preferential share in the game secured, but part of each catch is generally divided among the community among those present at the apportioning; (3) stored provisions are normally the property of the family or household, but in time of scarcity there is a tendency towards communalism. Hospitality is stressed under all circumstances. The Eskimo's dearest pastime is visiting. When someone has good catching or hunting he'll stand outside of his house and call out for people to come and visit him. Sometimes there may only be less than half a dozen families at the settlement, and they will all come to the house when he calls. When they come in he may ask if they want something to eat, as though it's an afterthought. Then

he will even describe how poor his catch was, that his wife is a poor cook, and that they must suffer not having very good food. In certain Eskimo areas, the larger feasts are not attended by women, although they do eat well. This sharing is something that helps prevent starvation and also helps make life happy and enduring.[11]

One of the strongest taboos in Eskimo societies was against eating a bear's liver. Stefansson said it was believed to be poisonous.[12] To test this belief, his group consumed a dozen polar bear livers. About a fifth of the livers made the men ill, causing bad headaches and vomiting. Stefansson speculated that the poisoning was due to a high level of some type of vitamins that were stored in the liver. At the time of his writing, he had little knowledge of the information that was available on vitamin A hypervitaminosis [see appendix C].

The customs and lives of these northern peoples have been influenced by contact with Western cultures. Snow tractors and motorized sleds are used to facilitate traveling long distances in place of dog sleds. Still present, however, is the Eskimos' heritage of living off the land in a subsistence lifestyle.

Notes

1. Peoples of the far north, like many of those encountered by Europeans during the age of exploration, do not refer to themselves by the names Europeans assigned them, though many have become resigned to the nomenclature. Some indigenous arctic peoples, however, reject the term "Eskimo" outright. Presently, in Canada, the people once assumed (by Europeans) to be virtually indistinguishable from Siberia to Greenland as Eskimos are known as Inuit. In northern Alaska, the resident group of these people are the Iñupiat; from Bering Strait to the northern shore of the Alaska Peninsula live the Yup'iks. Various Indian groups known as Athabaskans occupy the interior of Alaska and large parts of northern Canada. The indigenous people of Alaska who resided on the land before Bering's second voyage are collectively known as Alaska Natives; in Canada, they are members of the First Nations. In some instances, it is impossible to ascertain to which of these peoples an earlier source refers, and hence this text often falls back on the inept collectives "Eskimo" or "Indian."
2. B. Lopez, *Arctic Dreams, Imagination and Desire in a Northern Landscape* (New York: Charles Scribner's Sons, 1986), 7.
3. E. M. Weyer, *The Eskimos. Their Environment and Folkways* (Hamden, Ct.: Archon Books, 1962), 7.
4. Ibid., 2.
5. R. Fortuine, "Scurvy and its Influence on Early Alaskan History," *Arctic Medical Research, Supple* 1, 47 (1988): 311.
6. *Webster's Third New International Dictionary of the English Language Unabridged* (Springfield, Ma.: Merriam-Webster Inc., Publishers, 1993), 775.

7. V. Stefansson, *Not By Bread Alone* (New York: Macmillan Co., 1946), 38.

8. Ibid., 23.

9. F. Nansen, *The First Crossing of Greenland* (London: Longmans, Green and Co., 1892), 89.

10. E. M. Weyer, *The Eskimos, Their Environment and Folkways*, 115.

11. Ibid., 188.

12. V. Stefansson, *Not By Bread Alone*, 33.

5

Northern Exploration from 1500 to 1800

During the 16th, 17th, and 18th centuries many wars were fought in the western world. Interest in explorations of the polar areas fluctuated with successes and failures in war and with times of peace. Most of the expeditions were composed of relatively small numbers of men, although a few larger ones were attempted.

Many people became well known for their expeditions. Jacques Cartier sailed from Saint Malo, France, along the eastern coast of what is now Canada and followed the Saint Lawrence River to present day Quebec. In 1541 he reached the Charles River and the site of what is now Montreal. In 1576 to 1578 Sir Martin Frobisher, under the flag of England, became famous for bringing back "golden ore" which set off a scramble for gold.[1] John Davis from England sailed through areas around Greenland and Baffin Island from 1585 to 1586, leaving his name on Davis Strait. In 1585 to 1587 he sailed around Greenland and Labrador and later went to the South Pacific.

In 1594, Willem Barents of Holland sailed to what are now the Russian islands of Novaya Zemlya and modern Svalbard. Henry Hudson, sailing from England in 1609 through 1610, ended up in the Hudson Strait in Hudson Bay, his namesakes. From 1612 to 1616 William Baffin from England sailed around Greenland, Spitsbergen, Hudson Strait, and even over to Lancaster Sound. With Robert Bylot as his pilot, Baffin is credited for his descriptions of Eskimo habits and food.

Although all of the early explorers had some food problems during their expeditions, Jens Munk's were the most pitiful.[2] In an extensive diary Munk told the terrible tale, starting with two ships sailing from Copenhagen under a Danish flag during May of 1619.[3]

Forty-eight men were aboard his larger ship, the *Unicorn*, and sixteen aboard the smaller one, the *Lamprey*. Several men died of natural causes en route before reaching the ice. The expedition spent the winter at what is now the present site of Churchill in Hudson Bay. By New Year's Day most of the crew were still in good health. Although their supplies were greatly reduced, they had been able to shoot birds, and they had caught at least one fox. By March 21, 1620, general malaise and dysentery attacked the entire crew, and they began dying at the rate of one every few days. Their teeth had started to decay, and they had developed mouth problems. Although Munk was able to collect a few herbs and some berries, the berries deteriorated under the sunlight. The deaths continued. By May most were bedridden. When, at a later time, some were able to shoot some birds, they were unable to eat them and had to make extracts. On May 28, Munk noted in his diary:

> All the limbs and joints were miserably joined together with great pains in the loins as if a thousand knives had been thrust through them. The body was black and blue, as when one gets a black eye, and the whole body was quite powerless. The mouth was in a very bad and miserable condition, as the teeth were loose and they could not eat any victuals.[4]

Somehow some survived until June, when the three surviving crew members were able to get out and gather some roots and green materials. Soon they were able to catch some trout, and their health slowly improved. On July 16 the survivors were able to sail out in their smaller ship. Of the group that started, sixty-one of Munk's men had died. Although other diseases such as dysentery caused deaths, the major causes were general malnutrition and eventual severe scurvy.[5]

The members of this expedition, and others, were adventurers and they knew that they might encounter unknown dangers in the course of their travels. John Davis was killed in 1605 fighting Japanese pirates in the East Indies. Willem Barents died after being put to sea in an open boat when returning to Holland. In the most invidious event of all, Henry Hudson, his son, and some associates were never seen again after being set adrift in a small open boat by mutineers of his ship in his bay, Hudson Bay.

While explorations of the arctic seas were undertaken in the 16th, 17th, and 18th centuries, explorations of what is now the vast Canadian territory were also under way. They began just north of what is now the border of the United States and from what is now Quebec going from Hudson Bay west and north. By 1670 the grand Hudson Bay Company was formed. Under a royal charter it became a private but government-interrelated company. It was also a governing body that had the equivalent of its own army. During

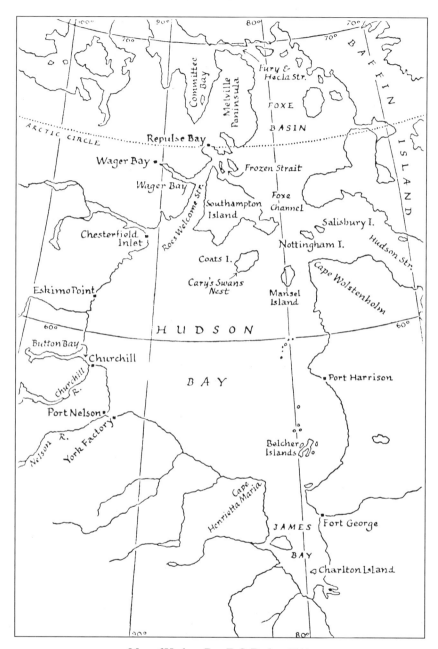

Map of Hudson Bay. E. S. Dodge, 1961

the intermittent conflicts with the French in the 1700s, members of the company stationed in outposts wore clothing that resembled uniforms, with officers wearing insignia on their caps. Possibly nothing was ever like it in the then-British empire other than the more grandiose East India Company. On the charts of organization held in London and in the operations in the main outposts, daily matters were conducted with thoughts to the rituals and codes of the Royal Navy.

Such administrative rules and restrictions, obviously considered necessary because of the distant enterprises, offered some stability and some acquiescence to authority. On the other hand, such rules inhibited the individuality and the freedom to act independently that so frequently was necessary for survival.[6]

Although it had many weaknesses, the Hudson Bay Company carried on a flourishing business, primarily trading in furs, initially firmly based on beaver pelts. Since it engaged in buying and selling products of the wilderness, it was responsible for extensive explorations, not only in the midcontinent but up to the polar coasts of the northern edge of the continent. Many who were associated with the Hudson Bay Company have given detailed insights into the foods, habits, and sicknesses of the explorers.

Seeking a northwest passage through the Hudson Bay, the *Dobbs Galley* and the *California* sailed from England in May of 1746 with William Moor and Francis Smith as leaders. They wintered by York Factory (of the Hudson Bay Company) and provide a vivid description of their experience suffering from scurvy:

> It is a melancholy, but withal a necessary task, to describe the progress of this fast and fatal distemper. Our men, when first seized with it, began to droop and grow heavy and at length indolent to the last degree: a tightness in the chest, pains in the breast, and a great difficulty in breathing, followed; then ensued livid contraction of the limbs, putrid gums upon the near back bone, with countenances bloated and fallow. These symptoms continually increasing, till at length, death carried them off, either by a flux or a dropsy. Those medicines, which in other countries are generally used with good effects, proved ineffectual here; the unctions and fomentations, when applied to contracted limbs afforded no relief, fresh provisions indeed, when we could get them, did somewhat, but the only powerful prevailing medicine, was tar-water, and the steady use of this saved many.[7]

Perhaps even more valuable was their description of the high antiscorbutic value of constantly consuming a drink that was called spruce beer. In the eyes of the Hudson Bay employees, spruce beer was superior to tar water. From as many as a hundred men at four different Hudson Bay installations, not a single man was buried over a seven-year period. This outcome is attributed to plentiful drinking of spruce beer. But they also reported that excessive drinking of strong spirits increased the incidence of scurvy.

Perhaps the most colorful of all Hudson Bay Company's explorers was Samuel Hearne.[8] The company sent him north and west to seek copper; his goal was to travel northwest to the Arctic Ocean at the Coppermine River. This took him across barren grounds and through difficult gravelly bogs en route to the frozen arctic shores. Starting in November of 1769 with two company employees and a pair of Cree hunters from the Prince of Wales fort, he was accompanied by a group of Chippewayan Indians. Two hundred miles away the Chippewayans turned on him and took every possession.

Hearne made it back to Prince of Wales fort, having learned in a very difficult way how to live off the land. In February of 1770 he was off again, only to be once more in the hands of the Chippewayans, who again took almost everything he had, leaving him in September, on the threshold of winter, without snowshoes, tents, or warm clothes. There would be no story about Hearne if he had not been joined by a Chippewayan chief named Matonabbe, who provided him with warm clothing and helped him develop the means to get back to Prince of Wales fort.

The friendly Matonabbe and Hearne then trekked off for the north, accompanied by Matonabbe's family of numerous wives and children. Off and on they were joined by other groups of Chippewayans, and Hearne adopted a native lifestyle. He ate everything the Indians ate except lice and warble flies. After four months Matonabbe and Hearne stopped to dry meat and build canoes. They were joined by another group of Indians. Only later did he understand that these were Copper Indians and that they were planning a raid on Eskimos at the mouth of the Coppermine River. The raid was a terribly bloody one, with extensive mutilations, rapes, and destruction. On July 18, 1771, Hearne was at the Arctic Ocean, on Coronation Gulf.

The return home took almost a year, but Hearne had completed a round trip of about 3,500 miles. He succeeded in completing the trip because he adopted the customs of the Natives. Although Hearne did not find a copper mine or a waterway to the northwestern arctic, he left a vivid description of his journey and of the people, the land, the animals, and some plants.

On his next expedition with Indians they fished with nets each day, which supplied their daily food. When fishing ceased to be successful, a hunter went out and "brought with him the blood and fragments of two deer that he had killed."[9] The expedition members wasted no time cooking a large kettle of broth made with the blood together with some fat and scraps of meat, shredded small, boiled in it. When food was unavailable, Hearne describes their effort to relieve their hunger:

> On those pressing occasions I have frequently seen the Indians examining their wardrobe which consists chiefly of skin-clothing and consider what part could best be spared; sometimes a piece of an old, half-rotten deer skin and in others a pair of old shoes were sacrificed to alleviate extreme hunger. The relations of such uncommon hardships may perhaps gain little credit in Europe; while those who are conversant with the history of Hudson Bay, and who are thoroughly acquainted with the distress which the natives of the country about frequently endure, may consider them as no more than a common occurrence of an Indian life, in which they are frequently driven to the necessity of eating one another.[10]

Of the many northern treks, Alexander Mackenzie's took place entirely over land (and, of course, rivers). In 1789 Mackenzie left Fort Chippewayan on Lake Athabaska with a small party of Canadians and Indians, hoping to follow a river to the Pacific Ocean. Instead he followed the great river that now bears his name, the Mackenzie River, to the Beaufort Sea, just east of what is now Alaska. He returned by the middle of October, having success-fully completed a 102-day trip without any serious incidents. On this trip he made many observations of Indian life, plants, and animals, relying on the birds, mammals, fish and plants of the areas he visited for food. His group killed many geese and deer; they frequently obtained liquorice root, wild parsnips, cranberries, and raspberries. As staples, he carried corn and pemmican, even caching it in the ground en route.

Three years later Mackenzie made his second trip, this one to the west coast across the Rocky Mountains. Leaving Fort Chippewayan in October of 1793, he followed rivers to the west with only one major overland trek. He reached the mouth of the Bella Coola river in Dean Channel on July 20, 1794. He was then convinced that there was no river-lake northwest passage across the northern continent to the Pacific Ocean. Mackenzie completed his explorations before the age of forty.[11] Fame as the first white man to cross the continent was not his only reward. Mackenzie became very wealthy as a fur trader and spent his last years at home in Scotland.

Notes

1. C. R. Markham, *The Lands of Silence* (Cambridge: Cambridge University Press, 1921), 85.
2. Farley Mowat, as an opinion, titled his description of the Munk expedition as "the black winter of Jens Munk."
3. See C. C. A. Gosch, ed., *Danish Arctic Explorations, 1605–1620,* Vol 2. 96, 97 (London: Hakluyt Society, 1897).
4. Ibid., 89.
5. Markham, *The Lands of Silence,* 151.
6. P. C. Newman, *Company of Adventurers* (Markham, Ontario: Penguin Books, Canada, Ltd., 1985), 3.
7. H. Ellis, *A Voyage to Hudson's Bay by the Dobbs Galley and California in the Years 1746–1747* (London: Whitridge, 1748). Tar-water was probably an infusion of parts of trees.
8. S. Hearne, *A Journey from Prince of Wales Fort in Hudson's Bay to the Northern Ocean* (Rutland, Vermont: Charles E. Tuttle Co., 1795).
9. Ibid., 24.
10. Ibid., 33.
11. A. MacKenzie, *A. Mackenzie, Voyages from Montreal on the River St. Laurence through the Continent of North America to the Frozen and Pacific Oceans in the Years 1789 and 1793 with a Preliminary Account of the Rise, Progress, and Present State of the Fur Trade of that Country* (London: R. Noble, Old-Bailey, 1801).

6

Arctic Exploration in the First Half of the 19th Century

The lure of money, fame, and excitement brought men to the Arctic and Antarctica. In the Arctic, men were often exposed to icy waters. In the antarctic, men were exposed to the swirling weather of the high plateau as well. In both polar areas, temperatures were frequently below -40°F (-40°C) with high winds and blizzards lasting for days. Frostbite of faces, hands, and feet was common. Even clothing presented a unique problem, becoming both heavy and stiff from frozen sweat. It was painful even to remove frozen socks and boots. Even simple tasks of voiding urine and feces could be painful.

On shipboard the climate made sailing and life both painful and perilous. Still, although men who sailed in both arctic and antarctic waters in the early 19th century suffered horrible polar storms, they did not suffer many of the life-threatening dangers encountered on polar lands. The ships usually survived the storms unless they were wrecked by collisions with icebergs or smashed by ice. It appears that the whalers were masters of avoiding such icy mishaps.

During the first half of the 19th century, both whaling and exploring accelerated in the arctic region. Whalers were motivated by an interest in discovering lucrative places to hunt. Unencumbered by the traditions and rules of the British navy and by British decorum, they ran wild and free. A prominent example of such a whaler was William Scoresby, who in 1806 went up north along the Greenland coast farther than anybody had gone before. Many of his trips produced no reports of nutritional problems, undue illnesses, or loss of life.

Among the many other polar explorers in the early 1800s, five stand out: William Edward Parry, John Ross, John Franklin, George Back, and James Clark Ross. Each achieved some fame in the Arctic or elsewhere.

In 1818 four British Royal Navy ships were sent north in two separate expeditions, one to sail to the pole via Spitsbergen and then to join the other to sail through the northwest passage. Both failed in their objectives, but the mission served as a polar training exercise for Franklin, Ross, and Parry, who were members of the expedition. Turned back after battering against the ice north of Spitsbergen, the two ships in which Franklin was a junior officer came home, worn and tattered. The other two were under the command of John Ross, with Parry as a junior officer. Although Ross made no new discoveries, he had a successful trip, with no undue losses. On return to England, however, there was a split between Parry and Ross. Parry accused Ross of mismanagement and was supported in his view by those at home, relegating Ross to the status of a poor explorer. Although this status was moderated by the the accomplishments of his later trips, Ross continued to be viewed as a minor figure in the history of exploration.

Parry made four more polar trips, achieving fame and even the rank of captain. Certainly, he was one of the great and most successful arctic explorers. In command at the age of thirty, Parry had already been in the navy for fifteen years. An accomplished leader, sailor, and navigator, he also was a talented actor and violinist, all of which aided his ability to improve the physical and mental health of his crews during the long arctic winters. In May of 1819 Parry made a deep thrust into Lancaster Sound.[1]

On this and on two more attempts to find a northwest passage, he was accompanied by James C. Ross, the young nephew of John Ross. On reaching 110° W latitude, the ships' crews received a monetary award of 5,000 pounds for their achievement. They wintered off Melville Island—1,200 miles west of Godhaven, Greenland, 700 miles north of a fur traders' post at Fort Providence on Great Slave Lake, and 1,200 miles east of Russian Alaska. They remained there during the winter, and good leadership carried them through; Parry balanced work with entertainment and made sure they had a proper diet.

Still, Parry had to make many unexpected adjustments. For one, the ration of freshly baked bread, a valuable food plus a morale builder, was necessarily reduced. Not only were the supplies limited, but the freezing of condensed moisture on the galley walls and ceilings precluded baking. Also, the stoves did not provide enough heat for baking. When lemon juice froze, it broke the bottles that contained it; the frozen contents would thaw and leak away. This also happened with kegs of vinegar, causing Parry to suggest that concentrated preparations of such items be taken in the future.

These problems combined with a lack of suitable warm clothing resulted in illness. By March twenty men were sick, half with scurvy. Parry broke out of the ice in August 1820 and returned to England with ninety-three of his original crew of ninety-four men.

Parry wasted no time in returning to the Arctic. In April of 1821, he set off with two ships, but this time to a more southern location, off Melville Peninsula (unrelated to Melville Island). Having learned from his previous experiences, Parry saw to it that his ships had better stoves. He grew cress and mustard on board to use in case of scurvy. He provided more entertainment and made some minor improvements in the clothing. This time the rations were well supplemented with seal, walrus, a little fish, and caribou. In October 1822 Parry again returned to England without much serious illness or other problems, although he did not make any new discoveries of value.

Unfortunately, his last attempt for the passage was catastrophic. One of Parry's ships, the *Fury*, was lost, but not before he was able to rescue some of the stores and provisions on board. He organized a depot of provisions on the shore, a depot that was eventually used by several later explorers. Parry ended his explorations by going forth again in 1827, endeavoring to reach the North Pole, crossing the land and ice by foot, man-hauling all the gear and provisions. This accomplished nothing except pain and suffering.

The British refused to use the Eskimo dog teams. Each man's daily ration included ten ounces of biscuit, nine ounces of pemmican, one ounce of sweetened cocoa powder, and one gill of rum. This ration did not meet the men's needs. Parry wrote: "Our daily allowance of provisions—proved by no means sufficient—an addition would be requisite of at least one third more to the provisions which we daily issued."[2] In the reports of Parry's expeditions, we must always consider the possible effect of the British admiralty to exploit the explorations of its officers. What was wrong in presenting them in the best of the high tradition of the navy, in other words, rewriting and reinterpreting reports?[3]

Although John Ross never obtained the good reputation that was probably due him and was shelved for his mismanagement, in 1829 he sailed again in a private expedition to locate the north magnetic pole and, possibly, to reach western waters.[4] James C. Ross was with him, now a commander under his uncle. John Ross did not obtain support from the admiralty but did obtain it from Felix Booth, a businessman (distiller) and sheriff of London. Unlike his previous expeditions, money was limited and the ship, the *Victory*, was very small. The ship could not accommodate more than meager stores, and the engine on the ship was totally inadequate, so Ross was reduced to sailing with a bare minimum of sail capacity.

One of his objectives was to obtain supplies from the wrecked *Fury* of the previous Parry expedition and, fortunately, he succeeded. Upon arriving at what was then called Fury Beach, the expedition members found the food depot in place and unspoiled. Cans of meats and vegetables were stored in two piles that had been exposed to all types of climate for four years. Apparently the cans were so solidly sealed that bears did not detect the contents, so all was left intact. The food was well preserved. Wine and other items, such as bread, flour, and cocoa, were in excellent condition, and even lime juice was among the supplies. All of these were critical for the eventual survival of the crew of the *Victory* to supplement their meager stores. Upon inventorying their provisions, they found enough for three years on full allowance, except for the wine. Ross thought that this was a benefit, however, because he believed that alcohol could increase the severity of scurvy.[5]

John Ross's expedition was exceptional, not only for its discoveries, but also for its leadership and management. Of the twenty-two men he had on board when he left England, nineteen returned with him after four years; only one man died from scurvy—all of this after abandoning the *Victory* and four long winters and the eventual rescue by another ship. One of his secrets had been to seek out fresh meat at every opportunity, and to befriend the Native inhabitants, obtaining their help to get fresh meat.

> It would be very desirable indeed if the men could acquire the taste for Greenland food; since all experience has shown that the large use of oil and fat meats is the true secret of life in these frozen countries, and that the natives cannot subsist without it; becoming diseased, and dying under a more meagre diet....I have little doubt, indeed, that many of the unhappy men who have perished from wintering in these climates, and whose histories are well known, might have been saved if they had been aware of these facts, and had conformed, as is so generally prudent, to the usages and experiences of the natives.[6]

The size of his group may also have had bearing on their success. It was small enough so that they could obtain sufficient food to live off the land. Still, Ross knew the terrible consequences of starvation, writing, "The scanty allowance of yesterday or today, the equal prospect of as scanty an allowance tomorrow, formed not matter for aught but serious thoughts, and even anxious care; it was not a question alone whether we should attain our object and execute our plans, but whether we should live or die."[7]

Never before had explorers lived for four straight winters in the arctic land. Never before had so much knowledge been obtained and with such a relatively small crew. Perhaps John Ross's success was a harbinger of Roald Amundsen's later huge success in navigating the polar route with a crew of only seven.

John Ross's homecoming stirred great interest throughout England, and his success brought into question the ability of the British admiralty to plan an expedition. Previously labeled an incompetent and undesirable person, Ross now had reestablished his honor. The admiralty was reluctant to acknowledge a different approach to arctic exploration, however. Planning could prevent problems such as scurvy, and even some from the wrath of the arctic climate, but human weaknesses could not be overcome. Sailors could still become disabled from drinking whiskey that was hidden on board, men could lose their minds, and starvation could lead to uncontrolled behavior. The British refused to admit that their inadequate winter clothing was so inferior to what the Scandinavians or Eskimos wore at that time. They believed that Eskimo food and the use of dogs were beneath a British sailor and certainly unthinkable for a British officer.

Some of these ideas persisted in further explorations into the Arctic. George Back, the commander of the *Terror*, followed in Parry's footsteps. Back's ship was beset by the icepack, drifted throughout the winter, and was badly damaged. He returned home, his ship a wreck and his men totally debilitated. Scurvy was rampant and three men died. None of the lessons that Ross learned were applied to prevent this type of disaster.

John Franklin was an old hand in the Arctic. He had sailed with John Ross and Parry in 1818. Then he commanded two land-based explorations. From 1819 to 1822 he was in command of the British arctic land expedition, leaving York Factory in Hudson Bay. The expedition wintered over and traveled northwest to reach the mouth of the Coppermine River. Although more or less following in Samuel Hearne's footsteps, they did not have Hearne's luck nor his expertise; many of the group died, two by murder and the rest from starvation.

Descending the Coppermine River, the expedition reached the polar sea successfully, but the return trip across land was disastrous, even ending in an execution. His group had to break into smaller units, some staying with ill companions, others seeking food or help. The threat of starvation was great. The men ate soup made of singed skin and bone and "made a sorry meal of an old pair of leather trousers and some swamp tea."[8] On a diet of such tea and no real food, they had serious problems with frequent urination. Franklin wrote, "the urinary secretion was exceedingly abundant, and we were obliged to rise from bed in consequence upwards of ten times a night."[9]

They were also faced with murder, cannibalism, and execution. Franklin reported these problems through Dr. John Richardson, a surgeon in the Royal Navy. The murderer and cannibal was an Indian named Michel. These actions were first suspected when Michel returned from a hunt. Richardson wrote,

> "He [Michel] reported that he had been in chase of some deer which passed near his sleeping-place in the morning, and although he did not come up with them yet, that he found a wolf which had been killed by the stroke of a deer's horn and had brought part of it. We implicitly believed this story then, but afterwards became convinced from circumstances, the detail of which may be spared, that it must have been a portion of the body of Belanger or Perrault."[10]

Missing is an acknowledgment that Richardson and the others also ate the meat, but they apparently did not suspect Michel of these activities as yet. Not too many days later, there was nearly conclusive evidence that Michel shot midshipman Robert Hood, and Richardson executed Michel.[11]

During their return trip they reached Fort Enterprise, only to find it unmanned and unstocked, and consequently experienced extensive malnutrition:

> Though the weather was stormy on the 26th, Samandré assisted me to gather tripe de roche [a lichen]. Adam, who was very ill, and could not now be prevailed to eat this weed, subsisted principally on bones, though he also partook of the soup. The tripe de roche had hitherto afforded us our chief support, and we naturally felt great uneasiness at the prospect of being deprived of it, by its being so frozen as to render it impossible for us to gather it.
>
> We perceived our strength declined everyday, and every exertion began to be irksome; when we were once seated the greatest effort was necessary in order to rise, and we had frequently to lift each other from our seats; but even in this pitiable condition we conversed cheerfully, being sanguine as to the speedy arrival of the Indians. We calculated, indeed, that if they should be near the situation where they had remained last winter, our men would have reached them by this day. Having expended all the wood which we could procure from our present dwelling without danger of its fall, Peltier began this day to pull down the partitions of the adjoining houses. Though these were only distant about twenty yards, yet the increase of labour in carrying the wood fatigued him so much that by the evening he was exhausted. On the next day his weakness was such, especially in the arms, of which he chiefly complained, that he with difficulty lifted the hatchet; still he persevered, while Samandré and I assisted him in bringing the wood,

Table 6.1

Probable basic ship provisions for Franklin expedition in 1845[a,b]

Day	Biscuit or flour (lb)	Saltbeef (lb)	Saltpork (lb)	Preserved meat (lb)	Sugar (oz)	Tea (oz)	Chocolate (oz)	Lemon juice (oz)
Monday	1	3/4	–	–	2 1/2	1/4	1	1
Tuesday	1	–	–	1/2	2 1/2	1/4	1	1
Wednesday	1	–	3/4	–	2 1/2	1/4	1	1
Thursday	1	–	–	1/2	2 1/2	1/4	1	1
Friday	1	3/4	–	–	2 1/2	1/4	1	1
Saturday	1	–	–	1/2	2 1/2	1/4	1	1
Sunday	1	–	3/4	–	2 1/2	1/4	1	1

a. Each man probably received in addition one pint of soup every week and oatmeal, vinegar, mustard, pepper, etc. as ordered.

b. From reconstruction by Cyriax (1939).

but our united strength could only collect sufficient to replenish the fire four times in the course of the day. As the insides of our mouths had become sore from eating the bone soup, we relinquished the use of it, and now boiled the skin, which mode of dressing we found more palatable than frying, as we had hitherto done.

On the 29th, Peltier felt his pains more severe, and could only cut a few pieces of wood. Samandré, who was still almost as weak, relieved him a little time, and I aided them in carrying in the wood. We endeavoured to pick some tripe de roche, but in vain, as it was entirely frozen. In turning up the snow in searching for bones, I found several pieces of bark, which proved a valuable acquisition, as we were almost destitute of dry wood proper for kindling the fire. We saw a herd of rein-deer sporting on the river about half a mile from the house; they remained there a long time, but none of the party felt themselves strong enough to go after them, nor was there one of us who could have fired a gun without resting it.[12]

Franklin made the next expedition from 1825 to 1827, and this time there were only a few problems. They were successful, even living partially off the land. Nevertheless, they had extensive support for supplies from the Hudson's Bay Company. After this, for a long time Franklin was the governor general of what is now Tasmania.

In 1845 the admiralty settled on a grandiose expedition and chose John Franklin to lead it. The goal was to sail across the northern arctic into the Bering Sea and to do geomagnetic work. The expedition was beset with problems.

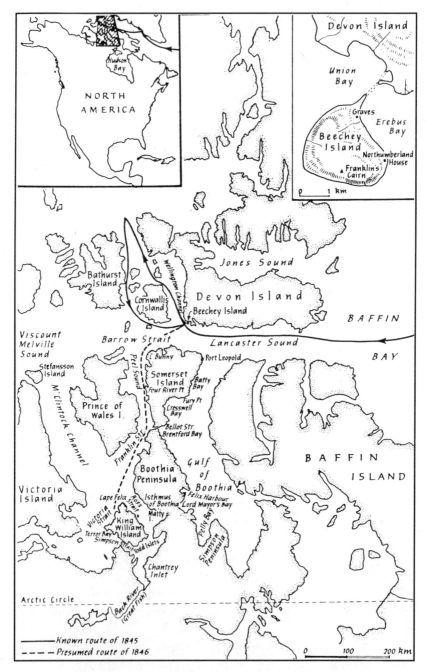

Route of the ill-fated Franklin expedition. O. Beattie and J. Geiger, 1987

At that time Franklin was fifty-nine years old, and too old for the job in the opinions of many. Pierre Berton believes that this very ambitious expedition was placed in the hands of Franklin because people felt sorry for him; this was to be his last big chance.[13] However, Franklin certainly had the experience and know-how, and he outfitted the expedition with the best of everything. At all times it was a British naval expedition. They had specially fitted ships, the *Erebus* and a rebuilt *Terror*, which had previous experience in Antarctica. In contrast to some of the earlier crews, this crew for Franklin was selected from what was considered the best of navy men on the basis of health as well as experience. There were 129 of them, and they had four solid years' worth of rations. All this equipment and experience, unfortunately, did not insure success. The last contact with them was when they hailed two whaling ships in Baffin Bay during July 1845. Everything else about them has been mainly obtained from scraps of information brought in by many individuals, including conversations with Eskimos.

Their first winter was at Beechy Island, where they were frozen in. Franklin, along with some others, died during that winter. At that time they apparently had nothing to do with the Eskimos, a beginning of their tragedy. Then the ships were abandoned by most of the crew, only a few men apparently staying with their ships.

The main documents about the expedition were a result of a later finding by Francis Leopold McClintock's search party. They were written by a man named F. R. M. Crozier, one of Franklin's lieutenants. He left a message on the northwest coast of King William Island, in which he wrote that they left on June 11, 1847, and had arrived at this point with 104 men after traveling thirty miles across treacherous sea ice. The two ships, *Erebus* and *Terror*, had been frozen in Victoria Strait for two years; Franklin and twenty-three others were dead. Crozier stated that he intended to lead the group 250 miles south and east to the mouth of Back's Fish River. From there he hoped to reach human habitation. Apparently a few returned to the ship, and Crozier's group was then split into two: forty went with Crozier towards the Back River and the others turned east. Somewhere around Cape Herschel Crozier and his men encountered four Eskimo families who gave them meat. But the Eskimos knew that they could not travel with the group because they could not feed their families and the Crozier men as well.

Crozier's people never appreciated this concept, and most all of the British experts up to that time did not know the importance of traveling in small groups. Only at the times when the great herds of caribou were

Table 6.2

Principal foodstuffs supplied for the H.M.S. *Erebus* and H.M.S. *Terror* for Franklin's expedition in 1845[a,b]

Foodstuff	H.M.S. *Erebus*	H.M.S. *Terror*	Total
Biscuit	18,355 lb	18,132 lb	36,487 lb
Flour	69,888 lb	66,768 lb	136,656 lb
Pemmican	612 lb	591 lb	1,203 lb
Beef in 8-lb pieces	16,416 lb	15,808 lb	32,224 lb
Pork in 4-lb pieces	16,320 lb	15,680 lb	32,000 lb
Preserved meat	16,066 lb	17,223 lb	33,289 lb
Sugar	11,928 lb	11,648 lb	23,576 lb
Preserved vegetables	4,572 lb	4,328 lb	8,900 lb
Concentrated spirits	1,896 gal	1,788 gal	3,684 gal
Wine for the sick	100 gal	100 gal	200 gal
Suet	1,568 lb	1,484 lb	3,052 lb
Raisins	504 lb	504 lb	1,008 lb
Peas	75 bus	72 bus	147 bus
		4 gal	4 gal
Chocolate	4,822 lb	4,628 lb	9,450 lb
Tea	1,195 lb	1,162 lb	2,357 lb
Lemon juice	4,750 lb	4,550 lb	9,300 lb
Concentrated soup equivalent to	10,920 pt	9,543 pt	20,463 pt
Vinegar	677 gal	649 gal	1,326 gal
Scotch barley	1,248 lb	1,248 lb	2,496 lb
Oatmeal	690 gal	660 gal	1,350 gal
Pickles	300 gal	280 gal	580 gal
Cranberries	85 gal	85 gal	170 gal
Mustard	500 lb	500 lb	1,000 lb
Pepper [c]	100 lb	100 lb	200 lb

a. These were the provisions for 129 men for three years.
b. From Cyiax (1939).
c. No mention is made of salt.

traveling, or when the fishing and sealing was plentiful (and these were short times), could large groups of people travel across the Arctic and obtain enough sustenance. After the meeting with the Eskimos apparently things worsened considerably, and members of the contingent continued to die. Finally the last thirty members of the group died.

Bits of evidence have shown that they hauled with them much material that was unnecessary and required much energy to carry. One of the items, a boat mounted on a sledge, was later found; it was estimated to weigh nearly three-quarters of a ton. They also carried silk handkerchiefs, two rolls of sheet lead, and twenty-six large silver spoons, forks, and teaspoons. Even some delftware teacups and officers' swords were found. No food was discovered, other than some tea and chocolate. The location of the discovery, which is near Barrow Inlet on Adelaide Peninsula, has been called Starvation Cove.

Over fifty expeditions during the next decade and a half were organized to search for Franklin, and hundreds of books or articles have been written on his disastrous expedition. Perhaps if Franklin had lived, or someone like Ross had been there to take Franklin's place when he died, a total loss of life may have been avoided. Over half a century later, Peary lamented about the disaster:

> Franklin's party, the largest in the history of polar exploration, equipped with everything that the ample resources of the British Government could provide in that day, met with disaster, not a single member surviving to tell the fate which overtook them. Too large a party was, in my opinion, the direct cause of the utter loss of this expedition, and many of the tragedies which have preceded and followed it would not have occurred had the parties been small ones.[14]

Notes

1. W. E. Parry, *Three Voyages for the Discovery of the Northwest Passage in 1819–20* (New York: Harper & Brothers, 1821). W. E. Parry, *Journal of a Second Voyage in 1821–23* (New York: Harper & Brothers, 1824). W. E. Parry, *Journal of a Third Voyage in 1824–25* (New York; Harper & Brothers, 1826). W. E. Parry, *Narrative of an Attempt to Reach the North Pole... in 1827* (New York: Harper & Brothers, 1828).
2. Parry, *Narrative of an Attempt to Reach the North Pole... in 1827*, 325.
3. Politics, economics of book publishing, or even affection of loved ones can be the cause of the modification of facts. John Rae complained that his book, *Narrative of an Expedition to the Shores of the Arctic Sea in 1846 and 1847*, "was so remolded that I did not know my own bantling when it reached me about three years after I left

England"; see P. C. Newman, *Company of Adventurers* (Penguin Books, Canada, Limited, Markham, 1986), 395. R. Huntford, commenting upon the information spread in Britain on the expeditions of Scott and Amundsen, wrote: "It was characteristic of Britain at the time that very few asked why Amundsen had succeeded. The most astonishing manipulations of acts were performed in order to prove that the British had not been worsted and, but for a little bad luck, all would have been well." See R. Huntford, *The Last Place on Earth* (London: Pan Books Ltd., 1985), 513.

4. J. Ross, *Narrative of a Second Voyage in Search of North-West Passage and a Residence in the Arctic Regions During the Years 1829, 1830, 1831, 1832, 1833* (London: A. W. Webster, 1835).

5. H. Ellis, *A Voyage to Hudson's Bay by the Dobbs Galley and California in the Years 1746–1747* (London: Whitridge, 1748).

6. J. Ross, *Narrative of a Second Voyage in Search of North-West Passage*, 201.

7. Ibid., 636.

8. J. Franklin, *Journey to the Shores of the Polar Sea in 1819-20-21-22*, Vol 4 (London: John Murray, 1829), 95 and 156. Swamp tea was probably an infusion of leaves of plants.

9. Ibid., 136.

10. Ibid., 102.

11. Ibid., 116.

12. Ibid., 89–90.

13. P. Berton, *The Arctic Grail* (New York: Viking Penguin, 1988).

14. R. E. Peary, *Secrets of Polar Travel* (New York: The Century Co., 1917), 44.

7

The Agonizing Searches
for Franklin

By the third year after the Franklin expedition's departure, strong fears ran through the people of England that the expedition had met with disaster. Plans were soon instituted for a rescue, and then, as time went on, for simply learning what had happened. Accusations, recriminations, and even suggestions of criminal actions were made against the administrators who had provided food and other support for the Franklin expedition.[1]

One person who was not a member of an expedition was soon to be accepted as a shining example of British fortitude, love, and unwillingness to admit defeat. This was Lady Jane Franklin.[2] She extolled the value of her husband's exploits and promoted exploration in her husband's behalf long after he died. It meant pounding on the doors of the admiralty for money, ships, and men to search for her husband and his shipmates, as well as raising money elsewhere and using her own resources in supporting future expeditions. She even wrote a letter to U.S. President Zachary Taylor, asking for American aid, which came in the form of two American brigs, the *Advance* and the *Rescue*.

When hope was still possible for finding members of the Franklin expedition alive, James C. Ross was commissioned by the admiralty to lead the search. In 1848 Ross's expedition left in two ships, the *Enterprise* and the *Investigator*. His lieutenants were Robert McClure and Francis Leopold McClintock. They mapped some of the land but found no sign of the Franklin expedition. Low morale from the lack of success and exhaustion from man-hauling poorly designed sledges plagued them. Nevertheless, they man-hauled their sledges for more than five hundred miles in thirty-nine days, unknowingly coming close to solving the Franklin mystery. On return to their ship, four out of twelve men were debilitated by inadequate rations. By the end of summer, all the men suffered from malnutrition. The

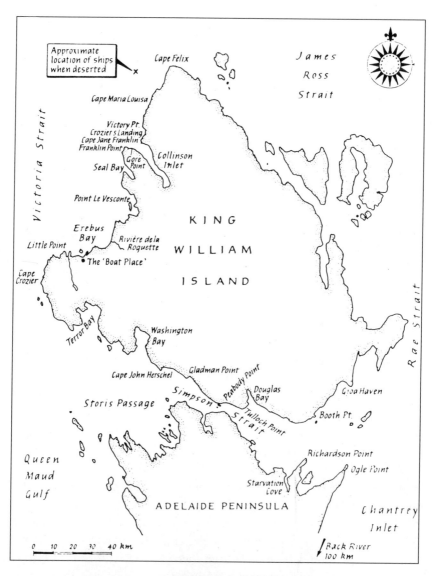

The end of the Franklin expedition at King William Island.
O. Beattie and J. Geiger, 1987

combination of exhaustion with the lack of fresh food brought on scurvy, which was rampant, and seven men died.[3]

In 1854 McClure and Richard Collinson sailed from Honolulu to go into the Arctic from north of Alaska. Collinson took the *Enterprise* through the western end of the Arctic and found a place where a northwest passage could be achieved. Hampered by the usual difficulties of the British Navy's commitment to man-hauling across ice, they made it by brute force but found no evidence to explain Franklin's disappearance. After being frozen in the ice and away from home for three and a half years, they returned to England.

It was on the 1848 expedition with Ross and McClure that McClintock learned and developed "the art of sledge travelling which he soon afterwards brought to such perfection."[4] Following a second search in 1850, McClintock commanded an expedition in July 1857 that was largely financed by Lady Franklin, and he was successful in his search for evidence of the Franklin party's fate.[5] He traveled on the *Fox*, a steam yacht of only 177 tons, eventually experiencing the usual drifting and freezing in the ice encountered in the Arctic. He found much of the evidence, including skeletal remains, on King William Island. On returning to England, McClintock received a hero's welcome and, after further duties in the Arctic and at home, he died "in harness" at the age of eighty-nine.[6]

The searches for Franklin were not always led by men with backgrounds in exploration. One search was led by John Rae, a surgeon of the Hudson Bay Company and probably the most knowledgeable wilderness traveler by far. Many consider him one of the leading explorers and discoverers of northern Canada. Rae undertook four arctic expeditions and was one of the main three people who mastered the Eskimo way of eating, dressing, and traveling. He lived off the land and did not carry tons of food, tents, and modern equipment. Rae even enjoyed greater success than Hearne and others because he was either almost always alone or with people he had trained. During his work he walked for a distance of 23,000 miles. A later strong supporter of his was Vilhjalmur Stefansson.[7]

Rae was adept at obtaining foods and getting his men to eat all parts of game. Deer blood was used to make soup and meat was only slightly cooked. Preparing for the winter in 1846, Rae and his crew killed 109 deer, a musk ox, 53 brace of ptarmigan, and one seal, as well as netting 54 salmon.[8]

In August of 1853 Rae returned to Repulse Bay with seven men, including two Eskimo interpreters. After wintering over, he was off again to the northwest, where he met some Eskimos who informed him that at a large river some way off, thirty-five or forty white men had starved to death. Here he found evidence of the Franklin expedition:

> In the spring, four winters past (1850), whilst some Eskimo families were killing seals near the north shore of a large Island named in Arrowsmith's charts King William Land, forty white men were seen travelling in company southward over the ice, and dragging a boat and sledges with them. They were passing along the west shore of the above island. None of the party could speak the Esquimaux language so well as to be understood; but by signs the Natives were led to believe the Ship or Ships had been crushed by the ice, and they were then going to where they expected to find some deer to shoot. From the appearance of the Men (all of whom with the exception of one officer, were hauling on the drag ropes of the sledge and were looking thin)—they were then supposed to be getting short of provisions, and they purchased a small seal or piece of seal from the natives... At a later date the same season, but previous to the disruption of the ice, the corpses of some thirty persons and some graves were discovered on the Continent, and five dead bodies on an island near it, about a long day's journey to the north west of the mouth of a large stream, which can be no other than Back's Great Fish River...Some of the bodies were in a tent or tents; others were under the boat which had been turned over to form a shelter, and some lay scattered about in different directions. Of these seen on the Island, it was supposed that one was an officer (chief) as he had a telescope strapped over his shoulders, and his double barrelled gun lay underneath him...
>
> There appears to have been an abundant store of ammunition... a number of telescopes, watches, guns, compasses, etc., all of which seem to have been broken up, as I saw pieces of these different articles with the natives, and I purchased as many as possible, together with some silver spoons and forks, an Order of Merit in the form of a star, and a small plate engraved 'Sir John Franklin, K.C.B.'[9]

At this site, Rae also believed he found evidence of cannibalism: "From the mutilated states of many of the bodies and the contents of the kettles it is evident that our wretched Countrymen had been driven to the dread alternative of cannibalism as a means of sustaining life."[10] This observation outraged the admiralty as well as the popular press, and the evidence was not accepted. In the 1800s in England and in America, it was believed that righteous men would rather die than resort to such an unspeakable practice.[11] Fortunately for the honor of the admiralty, John Franklin could not have participated in any cannibalism. He had died of illness on the ship before the group embarked on their southern route.

John Rae and his men received an admiralty award of 10,000 pounds for their efforts to explain the fate of the Franklin expedition. Lady Franklin and others objected to the award on the basis that the whole story was yet

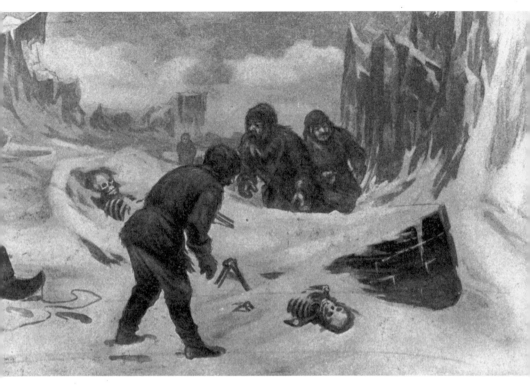

Finding of Franklin party by McClintock. C. Morris, 1909

unknown. Perhaps a few also objected because Rae was neither a navy man nor an aristocrat but a backwoodsman.

Confirmation of what Rae reported on cannibalism came much later from work done in the 1980s by Dr. Owen Beattie of the University of Alberta.[12] Beattie studied skeletal remains belonging to Franklin's sailors. He found evidence for scurvy and lead poisoning, as well as human bones that looked like a food supply because of evidence of saw marks due to human activity and other evidence of cut-up bodies.

Elisha Kent Kane, M.D., is another individual whose background was not typical of most explorers who searched for Franklin.[13] Kane was an excellent student but gave up his studies to join the U.S. Navy and travel the world. He even fought in the Mexican war in 1847. Kane went on the two Grinnell expeditions, so called because they were financed by Henry Grinnell, a New York shipping magnate. The expeditions were under special orders from the secretary of the U.S. Navy, the first to conduct an expedition to the arctic seas in search of Sir John Franklin and the second to extend the charts. On the first expedition, commanded by Lt. Edwin DeHaven, Kane went as the surgeon.[14] He was thirty years old. Kane commanded the second, and it was this expedition on which his reputation as a skilled explorer was established.

On the second expedition, Kane wintered at Rensselaer Harbor in northwest Greenland in 1853–1854 and again in 1854–1855.[15] During the second year that the ship was locked in the ice he enforced the antiscorbutic doses, made soup from the ship's rats (which synthesize large amounts of vitamin C), burned parts of the ship itself for heat, and rigged mirrors to throw sunlight into the holds where some men lay bedridden with scurvy. As a doctor he was apparently fairly successful in tending to the general welfare of his men. His description of problems with frozen foods reflect both accuracy and humor:

> All our eatables became laughably consolidated, and after different fashions, requiring no small experience before we learned to manage the peculiarities of their changed condition. Thus, dried apples became one solid breccial mass of impacted angularities, a conglomerate of sliced chalcedony. Dried peaches the same. To get these out of the barrel, or the barrel out of them, was a matter impossible. We found, after many trials, that the shortest and best plan was to cut up both fruit and barrel by repeated blows with a heavy axe, taking the lumps below to thaw. Saurkraut resembled mica, or rather talcose slate. A crowbar with chiseled edge extracted the lamina badly; but it was perhaps the best thing we could resort to.
>
> Sugar formed a very funny compound. Take q. s. of cork raspings, and incorporate therewith another q. s. of liquid gutta percha or caoutchouc, and allow to harden: This extemporaneous formula will give you the brown sugar of our winter cruise. Extract with the saw; nothing but the saw will suit. Butter and lard, less changed, require a heavy cold chisel and mallet. Their fracture is conchoidal, with hæmatitic (iron-ore pimpled) surface. Flour undergoes little change, and molasses can at -28° be half scooped, half cut by a stiff iron ladle.
>
> Pork and beef are rare specimens of Florentine mosaic, emulating the lost art of petrified visceral monstrosities seen at the medical schools of Bologna and Milan: crow-bar and handspike! for at -30° the axe can hardly chip it. A barrel sawed in half, and kept for two days in the caboose house at +76°, was still as refractory as flint a few inches below the surface.[16]

On and off the expedition members suffered from near starvation. On his first trip, as well as his second, Kane's medical skills were put to good use. Both his descriptions of the symptoms of scurvy and his medications are typical of the times:

An increased disposition to scurvy shows itself. Last twelve cases of scorbutic gums were noted at my daily inspections. In addition to these, I have two cases of swelled limbs and extravasated blotches, with others less severely marked, from the same obstinate disease. The officers too, the captain, Mr. Lovell, and Mr. Murdaugh, complain of stiff and painful joints and limbs, with diarrhea and impaired appetite: the doctor like the rest. At my recommendation, the captain has ordered an increased allowance of fresh food, to the amount of two complete extra daily rations per man, with potatoes, saurkraut, and stewed apples; and we have enjoined more active and continued daily exercise, more complete airing of bedding, &c. I have commenced the use of nitro-muriatic acid, as in syphilitic and mercurial cases, by external friction.

The state of health among us gives me great anxiety, and not a little hard work. Quinine, the salts of iron, &c., &c., are in full requisition. For the first time I am without a hospital steward.[17]

Later in the season he still attributed cures to hydrochloric acid as well as to saurkraut and lime juice:

With these cheering signs of returning warmth came a sensible improvement in my cases of scurvy. I ascribed it in a great degree to the free use of saurkraut and lime-juice, and to the constant exercise which was enforced as part of our sanitary discipline. But I attributed it also to the employment of hydrochloric acid, applied externally with friction, and taken internally as a tonic. The idea of this remedy, hitherto, so far as I know, unused in scurvy, occurred to me from its effects in cachectic cases of mercurial syphilis. I am, I fear, heterodox almost to infidelity as to the direct action of remedies, and rarely allow myself to claim a sequence as a result; but according to the accepted dialectics of the profession, the Acid. chlorohyd. dilut. may be recommended as singularly adapted to certain stages of scorbutus.[18]

Only through the provision of limited acquisitions of fresh meat did they survive. Since Kane was ill with rheumatic fever before sailing, the initial provisions had been inadequate. Salt meat was aboard, but no fresh or canned meat. For a while, the chief antiscorbutic consisted of gratings from raw potatoes, a food item he adamantly prescribed:

At dinner as at breakfast the raw potato comes in our hygienic luxury. Like doctor-stuff generally, it is not as appetizing as desirable. Grating it down, leaving out the ugly red spots and adding oil as a lubricant, it is as much as I can do to persuade the men to shut their eyes and bolt it, like Mrs. Squeer's molasses at Dotheboys Hall. Two absolutely refuse to taste it.[19]

In spite of his excellence in handling the nutritional problems, Kane still found it difficult to make treaties with the Eskimos in order to get food. He studied and adopted the ways of the Eskimos, and he and his people ate raw seal and walrus meat, wore furs, used dog sleds, and lived in igloos. By age thirty-four, Kane was a national hero. He died at the age of thirty-six.

Charles Francis Hall, another American, felt he had a mission to continue the search for Franklin that by 1860 had been abandoned by everyone else.[20] He obtained meager support and a very poor stock of supplies. His first attempt failed, but he tried again. Finally, after working his way up north, he was wrecked off Baffin Island, where he remained for two years. Working and exploring, even with a lack of equipment, he kept going. His success is due to the fact that he went to the Eskimos. He is credited with being the first white man who traveled with only Eskimos. Some say he was probably the first white man who adopted an Eskimo lifestyle. Although he found some information on the Franklin expedition, he did not make any major discoveries. Yet he did make a very important contribution by demonstrating that the problem of living in the far north could be surmounted by adopting the Eskimo lifestyle.

His second expedition was a five-year journey to the area where the Franklin party perished. This trip was an outstanding success. Discontent among the men and some scurvy occurred, but five years was a long time for such isolation. Hall made his third and final expedition in 1871. All he had was a converted U.S. Navy tugboat, which again went up through Baffin Bay trying to reach the North Pole. The journey was not well planned and doomed to failure. He and his crew had a long voyage. When they finally reached their winter berth in what came to be called Hall Basin, Hall died. Although clearly authenticated proof does not exist, some believe that he died of arsenic poisoning at the hands of his crew, probably being fed moderate quantities of arsenic in his food. Certainly, he died with some symptoms resembling arsenic poisoning. On this last trip, he gathered a crew of mixed nationalities who were largely without proper experience. Hatreds developed and his role as commander was severely weakened.

Historians have not paid as much attention to Hall as to Kane. Some of the notes from Hall's expeditions were important, however, as they describe Eskimos in the area and their interaction with the sailors.[21] For example, a ship picked up nine men from a whale boat on August 7, 1860, off Baffinland Coast. These nine men abandoned their ship due to poor management and particularly because of poor food. One man made a sworn document about some of their activities: on August 20 one man died and his companions cut him up and ate him. A few days later another man was attacked and the attacker was knifed, dying the following morning. His comrades cut him up and ate him. With no other food they soon ate their boots, belts, and any types of skins or animal materials they had with them. Finally they were found and saved by another ship on the 29th. The story illustrates what could, and did, happen when men were alone, without hope, and starving.[22]

About the same time as Hall was leaving for the Arctic, Dr. Isaac Hayes, a former arctic comrade of Kane, was returning from the Arctic.[23] Hayes and Kane, both physicians, had developed an animosity towards one another (a frequent occurrence for polar explorers). Besting Kane was probably an objective of Hayes.[24] Hayes left in July of 1860 with a small ship and a contingent of eighteen men, a number only a little larger than ten percent of Franklin's. Traveling north between Greenland and Ellesmere Island, Hayes hoped to prove that there was an open polar sea. He did not find a sea, but thought he had, and held to that belief to the day of his death twenty years later. Living in part off the land and using Eskimos to help him, his losses were small and problems few. Still, in his main effort to reach his dreamed-of open polar sea, he was defeated not just by the awesome masses of ice but also by a shortage of food.

Over fifty separate expeditions from several nations went into the Arctic hoping to find Franklin, or at least to solve the mystery of his disappearance. Even today, the overall reason for the disastrous fate of Franklin's expedition continues to be a question despite research on frozen corpses.[25] Based on examination of the sailors' remains, lead poisoning has been suggested, with the culprit being, of course, the sealing of the cans of food with solder.[26] But a caveat appears because most of the expedition members had unquestionably been exposed to high levels of lead throughout their preexpedition lives and may have had some residues of lead in their bodies.

Notes

1. People speculated that the canned food caused the deaths, and thus canning foods became a very unpopular method of preservation. See S. Thorne, *The History of Food Preservation* (Cumbria, England: Parthenon Publication Group, Kirkby Lonsdale , 1986), 40; and J. C. Drummond and A. Wilbraham, *The Englishman's Food, of Sir Jack Drummand, Dec'd* (Oxford: England: Alden Press, 1958).

2. The loss of the Franklin expedition cut into the bone of almost every Englishman. Many stories, some true and some not, circulated, and many poems and sea ditties were penned and sung. From the most dismal pub to the most fashionable club, songs were sung with reverence and hope.

3. C. R. Markham, *The Lands of Silence—A History of Arctic and Antarctic Explorations* (New York: The MacMillan Co. and Cambridge: Cambridge University Press, 1921), 248.

4. Ibid.

5. Ibid., 249.

6. L. McClintock, *The Voyage of the 'Fox' in the Arctic Seas* (London: John Murray, 1860).

7. C. R. Markham, 278.

8. Noting the ridiculous antipathy towards Rae, Stefansson quoted something that a Royal Geographical Society officer had said to the polar explorer, Ernest Shackleton, "Of course, anybody can succeed if he's willing to go native"; R. C. Newman, *Company of Adventurers* (Markham, Ontario: Penguin Books, Canada, Ltd., 1986), 194. In this short sentence is the essence of the reason for the failures of so many explorers at that time. Very few of the tools of today's civilized world were useful in the Arctic. Fuel-driven snow tractors, radios or airplanes, much less scientific knowledge of nutrition, did not exist. Dogs, igloos, native clothes, and native foods were available, however. If anything, the Eskimo diet was superior to that of the British for warding off scurvy.

9. E. E. Rich, A. M. Johnson, J. M. Wordie, and R. J. Cyriax, *John Rae's Correspondence with the Hudson's Bay Company on Arctic Exploration* (London: The Hudson's Bay Record Society, 1953), 274.

10. Ibid., 276.

11. In his weekly journal, *Household Words*, Charles Dickens furiously and perhaps even viciously attacked the idea that British seamen would engage in such an activity. See C. Dickens, "The Lost Arctic Voyagers," *Household Words* 245 (Dec. 2, 1854): 361–365.

12. O. B. Beattie and J. M. Savelle, "Discovery of human remains from Sir John Franklin's last expedition," *Historical Archaeology* 17, 2 (1983): 100–105; R. Amy, R. Bhatnagar, E. Damkjar, and O. Beattie, "The Last Franklin Expedition: Report of a Postmortem Examination of a Crew Member," *Can Med Assoc J* 135 (1986): 115–117; O. Beattie, and J. Geiger, *Frozen in Time* (Saskatoon: Canada: Western Producer Prairie Books, 1987).

13. E. K. Kane, *The U.S. Grinnell Expedition in Search of Sir John Franklin: A Personal Narrative* (New York: Harper and Brothers Publ., 1854).

14. Ibid.

15. E. K. Kane, *Arctic Explorations, The Second Grinnell Expedition in Search of John Franklin, 1853, 1854, 1855* (Philadelphia: Childs and Peterson, 1856).

16. Kane, *Arctic Explorations*, 63.

17. Kane, *The U.S. Grinnell Expedition*, 304.

18. Ibid., 325.

19. F. Mowat, *The Polar Passion* (Boston: Little, Brown and Co., 1967), 64. Potatoes are eaten by many today, but they are usually not considered an important part of a diet. In Ireland, and other parts of Europe over a century and a half ago, potatoes were a major part of their diet and an important source of vitamin C, a major contributor to good nutrition. As a boy, I learned the value of a potato from family stories of my paternal great-grandparents' flight from Ireland to escape the potato famine. They brought my grandfather to Boston, only to have my great-grandmother die in Boston harbor, the victim of disease resulting from malnutrition, probably including scurvy. Ireland had been hit particularly hard by the plant disease that killed the potatoes.

20. C. F. Hall, *Arctic Researches and Life Among the Esquimaux, Being the Narrative of an Expedition in Search of Sir John Franklin, in the Years 1860, 1861, and 1862* (New York: Harper and Brothers, 1865).

21. C. Loomis and M. A. Wilson, *The Story of Charles Francis Hall, Explorer* (New York: Alfred Knopf, 1971); P. Berton, *The Arctic Grail* (New York: Viking Penguin, 1988).

22. F. Mowat, *Ordeal by Ice* (Toronto: McClelland and Stewart Ltd., 1976), 342.

23. I. I. Hayes, *The Open Polar Sea: A Narrative of Discovery Towards the North Pole* (New York: Hurd and Houghton, 1867).

24. N. Fogelson, *Arctic Exploration and International Relations 1900–1932* (Fairbanks: University of Alaska Press, 1992), 14.

25. O. Beattie and J. Geiger, *Frozen in Time.*

26. "Lead Solder: Source of Body Lead in the Franklin Burials," *Nutrition Reviews* 48, 7 (1990): 292.

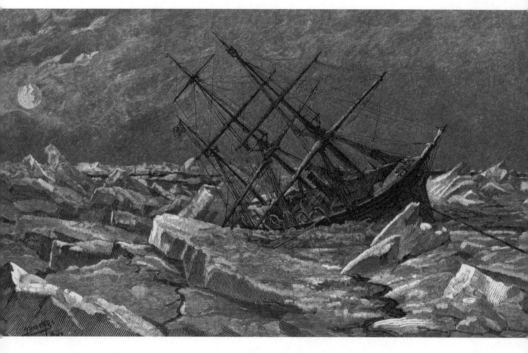

An example of how a ship was sunk by the ice. The sinking of DeLong's *Jeannette* in 1880.
E. DeLong, 1883

Nares, Greely, and DeLong: Still Unsuccessful and Tragic Probes to the North

For a few years after the intense searches for the Franklin expedition ended, there was a comparative lull in arctic explorations. The American Civil War and affairs in Europe were higher priorities. By the mid-1870s, there was a revival of interest in the Arctic.

In this revival Her Majesty's government ordered the British Navy to resume England's conquest of the north polar regions. The orders did not include many changes in the methods used on the expeditions, however, other than the addition of a few Eskimos and a very few dogs. For one of these new ventures Captain George Nares was commissioned to take a squadron of two ships, the *Alert* and the *Discovery*, through Baffin Bay and then to ram the ships north, going by land, if necessary, towards the North Pole.[1] Nares was not like most of the other leaders of polar expeditions. He was a career navy man, a nonexplorer, who did his duty as ordered. For him this was just another challenging job. On the way north he and his men killed musk oxen to supplement their rations, and the expedition was equipped and supplied for two full years.

The *Alert*, under Nares' leadership, went into winter quarters near Cape Sheridan on Ellesmere Island while the *Discovery* went into winter quarters on the north shore of Lady Franklin Bay. Several parties from the *Alert* went north on land, accomplishing much worthwhile mapping, including setting a new world's record for reaching the highest north-latitude point to that date. An unfortunate outcome of the journey was that nearly half of the 120 men came down with scurvy severe enough to incapacitate and nearly cripple them. The physical demands on the men were too great; the diet and the clothing was not adequate to ensure their good health.

Even though he must have known that man-hauling required much energy, on the sledgings Nares started with a daily ration of three-quarters of a pound of salt meat. Although he later increased it to a pound, this still did not meet the crew's energy and protein needs. He also should have known that their diet could not be supplemented with fresh meat, because animals would not be available to hunt.

Ship rations included four ounces of preserved vegetables, one ounce of which was pickled, and one pound of meat, which varied from day to day from sources that were salted or canned. They still had some fresh meat. It is not known how much juice was consumed, or whether the juice came from lemons or limes, or even if it was taken on sledging ventures at all.

At the end of the first winter, almost the entire crew had scurvy, and four men died from disease or accidents. Upon Nares' return to England, an inquiry was made into the accusation that as commander, he was responsible for letting his men get scurvy in one year. Many ideas were advanced as to what happened, but these did not include the real cause of the problem—the nutritional deficiency of the food. Debate continued over whether lime or lemon juice was really an antiscorbutic. Compounding the problem was that lemon or lime juice was stored in bottles that broke when the juice froze, and the contents would melt away. Thawing the juice was often inconvenient. This led to the suggestion that the juices should be dried. Nares believed that salted meat might contribute to the disease and recommended that it should never be supplied for polar expeditions. His observations may have helped the British Navy gain a little better picture of some of the nutritional problems experienced by expedition members.

The British military was not alone in dealing with nutritional difficulties in the Arctic. The explorations of two Americans, Army Lt. Adolphus Washington Greely and Navy Lt. George Washington DeLong, met with horrible disasters, both suffering from starvation. These expeditions had their roots in a hopeful gesture toward international scientific cooperation. In 1882 eleven countries established arctic stations for a year of observation. This became known as the First International Polar Year—the forerunner of two more, including one in the 1950s, which gave the final thrust to the extensive opening of Antarctica. One purpose of the first polar year program was to establish at Lady Franklin Bay a polar station, one of thirteen to make simultaneous observations of all possible physical phenomena. A station further to the north at Fort Conger was an American one commanded by Adolphus Washington Greely.[2]

Greely was a veteran of the Civil War, fighting in some of the bloodiest battles, rising from a seventeen-year-old volunteer to a brevet major. His later experience as a Signal Corps officer led to an interest in climatology

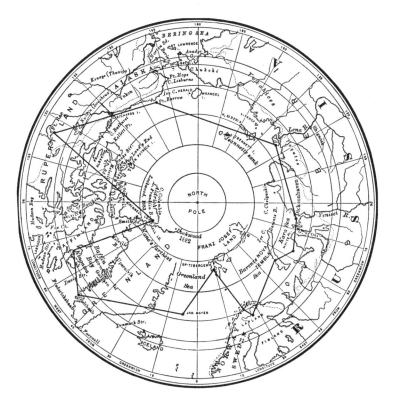

Map of arctic circumpolar stations (1881–1883), First International Program.
A. W. Greely , 1886

and he was selected to command the station in the Arctic. This command proved disastrous but did not end his career. He went on to command the U.S. Army's military governorship of San Francisco after the 1906 earthquake and then the incident of the Ute Indian rebellion (without bloodshed). Ronald T. Reuther has recently described him as "perhaps the foremost example of the small, but important, group of soldier-scientist-adventurers who led the nation into the 20th century."[3]

Greely's group was composed of three army officers, one acting assistant surgeon, and nineteen enlisted men selected from the ranks of the army on the basis of their having received high recommendations. Stores for twenty-seven months for the party were put on their ship, the *Proteus*. At Disco Island and Upernivik they procured sleds, dogs, skins, and dog food; two Eskimos were added later. They sailed up to Discovery Island and established a station at a site earlier occupied by the English Nares

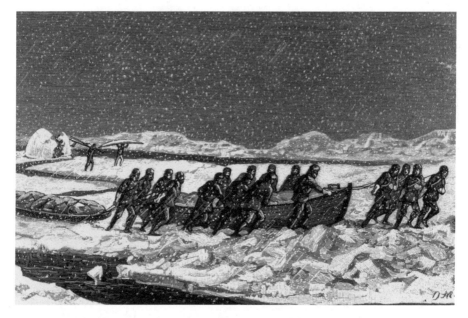

Fighting for life and boat in the Arctic. The crushing of the floe with the Greely party,
September 26, 1883. A. W. Greely, 1886

expedition of 1875. On August 28 Greely divided the crew into two parties,
one to travel by land, and the other to remain on ship. Greely led the land-
bound group of twenty-five men. He planned to establish a base camp and
explore on land for two years, then rendezvous with the ship and return
home. Only six of this group, including Greely, were alive at the end, after
being isolated for a third year. One man was executed, but the rest died of
misadventure or disease.[4]

Like so many arctic debacles, it was a tale based on bad food. When a
resupply ship did not come after a year, Greely and his men left their base in
August of 1882 and went south to Cape Hawks in two open boats and a
steam launch to search for food. Cape Hawks was the site of an English
depot from a former expedition. Greely found 342 pounds of stearine (a
lard), about 6 gallons of rum, 168 pounds of preserved potatoes, about 250
pounds of bread, and 10 gallons of pickled onions. Much had spoiled. The
bread was in casks and contained masses of green, slimy mold; some deemed
edible was extracted. The barrels and casks were broken up and taken for
steaming purposes. The food did not last for long, however, and crew
members considered other sources. They dredged for mussels and tried to

catch shrimp.[5] They caught a few birds. Their diet was not adequate to maintain good health, nonetheless, and men throughout the group were ill. One of the men, Lieutenant Lockwood, said "Our present ration is so small… it remains to be seen what the effect of any further reduction will be. We are hungry all the time. We have various seal skin articles of clothing which we talk of eating."[6] In camp, stealing food became a serious problem, and one man was executed for committing this crime.[7]

Greely, against the advice of others, began to add lichens to the diet, usually adding them to hoosh (stew). And so they tried tripe de roche. It had little or no taste because it was dry, but they considered it nutritious. Greely wrote, "I crawled on the rocks today, and got a can full of tripe de roche, half a pint. Some reindeer moss was also found. Had trouble from slight diarrhea from tripe de roche but still thought important."[8]

Greely issued to the party his seal skin jumper which had been reserved for shrimp bait. "I was able to eat very little of mine but ate instead about an ounce or two of boiled lichens which I had saved. Also cut off the dirty, oil tan covering of my sleeping bag and divided it among the party so that each man could have his part as desired."[9]

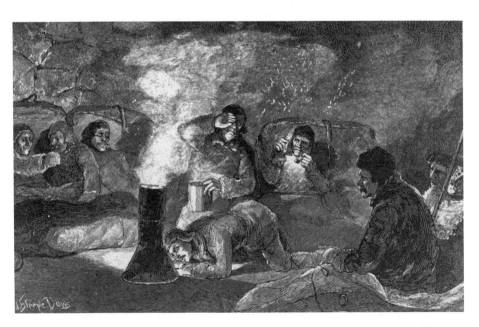

One of the better dinner times of arctic explorers in 1883. Interior of a winter hut of the Greely party at Camp Clay during cooking. A. W. Greely, 1886

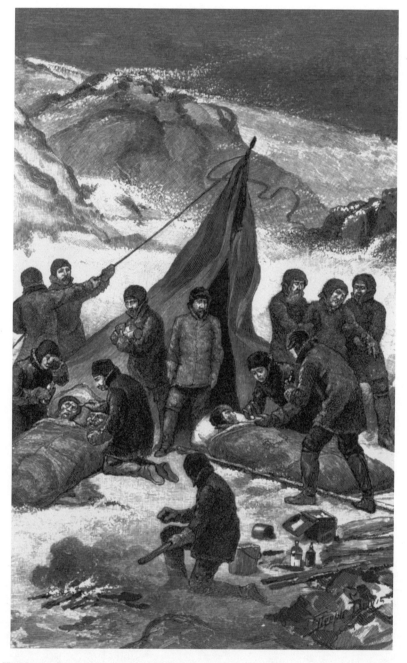

The finale of a terrible experience. The rescue of starving survivors of the Greely party,
June 23, 1884. A. W. Greely, 1886

On June 22, 1884, the remnants of the Greely party were rescued by the ship *Thetis*, under the command of a U.S. naval officer, Winfield Scott Schley. After they were rescued the adjutant general's office issued a report dated November 14, 1884, exonerating Greely for the execution of one of his men by saying that it was a necessary act in the performance of his duties.[10]

Many discussions, articles, and tabloid newspaper stories followed, most concerning the performance of Greely and his men. Cannibalism was frequently mentioned. Some of these comments came from interviews with survivors of the Greely party, but mainly with sailors of the rescue ship. One such example is from Schley's *The Bodies Were Mutilated*:

> In handling the remains after they had been prepared by the officers, the exceeding lightness of some of them was remarked upon by the seamen, and a doubt was more than once expressed if more than half of a body was within the covering. This was noticed in removing the bodies from their shallow graves in the gravel at the Cape and again when they were placed in the tanks on the *Bear* and *Thetis*—six in one and seven in the other. It is said that the body of the Esquimaux was not mutilated to any extent, but it was with reluctance that it was left at Disco, and then only by the imperative order of the inspector of Western Greenland. At Godhaven the Governor wished the body left, but he was prevailed upon to leave it with the others. At Disco, however, the demand for the remains was imperative. Some of the men had been little more than skin and bones when they died, but the little flesh they had was gone in some places, as on the calves of the legs, on the hips, thighs and arms. Some of this, it was asserted, was used as bait for shrimps, some to sustain the wasting life of the survivors. There seems, from the condition of the bodies, that there was no concerted action on the part of those remaining to sustain life in this way. None of the limbs were missing. But rather it seems that the perishing men went to the bodies when hunger became unbearable and supplied themselves as best they could.
>
> The disclosure made by unearthing the bodies of the dead was generally discussed by the crews of all the vessels on the homeward trip. Giving due allowance for the imagination of the sailors, the hard facts of the few who saw the remains and related what they saw to others before silence was enjoined, show that terrible scenes must have been enacted by the famishing men in the Greely camp during the many long months that famine was with them.[11]

Cannibalistic atrocities may have occurred during the Greely tragedy, but under other equally terrible circumstances, such as during the *Jeannette* expedition, cannibalism was not reported.

The *Jeannette* expedition was led by Lt. George Washington DeLong, a United States naval officer, who believed that he could reach the pole from what is now Russian territory, Wrangel Island. Of course, as we now know, Wrangel Island was not a large land mass that protruded far into the Arctic,

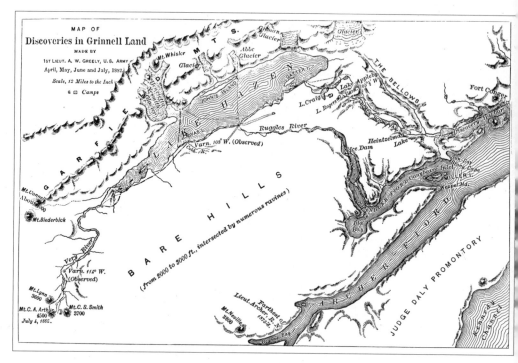

Map of Grinnell's discoveries in Grinnell Land. A. W. Greely, 1886

as Delong believed, and neither it nor other land masses would be an easy stepping stone to the pole. Delong's plan was supported enthusiastically by James Gordon Bennett, the owner of the *New York Herald*.[12]

In the summer of 1879 DeLong organized a thirty-two-man crew of misfits. Not believing in the superstition of sailors that changing a vessel's name brings bad luck, he purchased an old arctic ship and renamed her the *Jeannette*; it was outfitted in the San Francisco Naval Yard at Bennett's expense. DeLong ignored the shipyard workers' cautions that the *Jeannette* would not be suitable for foraging into the high polar waters.

After picking up two Eskimo hunters, the expedition members cruised through the Bering Strait into the Chukchi Sea, towards Wrangel Island. They were soon beset in the ice pack. The ship drifted for twenty-two months until June 1881 when finally the pressure of the ice crushed the ship and forced the crew to abandon it. They headed south in three open boats towards the New Siberian Islands. At this time they started with the following daily rations:

Breakfast	Dinner	Supper
4 oz. pemmican	8 oz. pemmican	4 oz. pemmican
1 oz. ham	1 oz. Liepig	1 oz. tongue
3 pieces bread	1/2 oz. tea	1/2 oz. tea
2 oz. coffee	2/3 oz. sugar	2/3 oz. sugar
2/3 oz. sugar	--	1 oz. lime juice
		1/4 lb. bread[13]

This would have supplied sufficient calories if all had gone well, with some dogs for hauling and a motor launch for pulling, but everything went wrong. These rations did not meet the nutritional needs of the men from the start, and their physical condition declined; some suffered from lead poisoning caused by the canned food. They did not have adequate clothing, not even boots that were appropriate for this type of march. They had to haul three boats in order to cross open waters. They had dogs but did not know how to use them properly. After a month of hauling by foot, they reached the coast. Here a disastrous separation occurred: one boat with DeLong and his fellow passengers went one way, a second boat disappeared

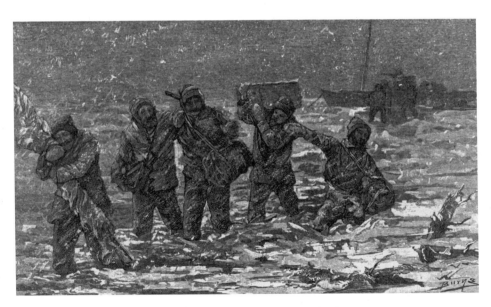

Wading ashore in the Arctic. E. DeLong, 1883

Table 8.1

The distribution of weights among five sleds on the *Jeannette* expedition. From *The Voyage of the Jeannette*, Vol. 2 (1883)

No. 1	No. 2	No. 3	No. 4	No. 5
765 lbs. Pemmican	720 P.	720 P.	720 P.	720. P
40 gallons Alcohol	40 A.	40 A.	40 A.	40 A.
36 lbs. Liebig	36 L.	—	—	18 L.
61 lbs. C. L. Sugar	—	—	—	61 S.
60 lbs. X. C. Sugar	—	—	—	—
4 bags Bread	4 B.	4 B.	4 B.	2 B. Br.
30 lbs G. Coffee	30 Coff.	—	30 R. Coff.	—
90 lbs. Tea	—	—	60 G. Coff.	—
10 lbs. X. C. Sugar	—	—	—	—
Total = 1,659 lbs.	1,318 lbs.	1,252 lbs.	1,342 lbs.	1,325 lbs.

On the ice yet 30 lbs. roast coffee, 30 lbs. ground coffee, 1 bag bread which must go in the boats. Still short of sixty days' provisions, viz.: 315 lbs. pemmican, 43 lbs tea, 55 lbs. sugar, 37 lbs. coffee.

without a trace, and a third, led by Chief Engineer George Melville, reached land. Melville guided it up the Lena River Delta where he was soon in contact with Natives. Out of the original thirty-two-man crew of the *Jeannette* expedition, only thirteen from Melville's group survived.

Melville, in his book, *In the Lena Delta*, describes the search for his lost shipmates.[14] In that search, with the help of a party of Natives, he and his group found the dead members of the DeLong expedition and buried them. They also found a diary record of DeLong's final march:

> Friday, October 7, 1881: The undermentioned officers and men of the late U.S. steamer *Jeannette* are leaving here this morning to make a forced march to Kumarksurt or some other settlements on the Lena River. We reached here on Tuesday, October 4, with a disabled comrade, H. H. Erickson, seaman, who died yesterday morning and was buried in the river at noon. His death resulted from frostbite and exhaustion due to consequent exposure. The rest of us are well but have no provisions left, having eaten our last this morning. Signed: George W. DeLong, Lieutenant Commanding, et al.
>
> October 7: Breakfast consisted of our last one-half pound of dog meat. Our last grain of tea was put in the kettle this morning and we are now about to undertake our journey of some twenty-five miles with some old tea-leaves and two quarts of alcohol [alcohol was used for energy].
>
> October 11: One teaspoonful glycerine and hot water for food. No more wood in our vicinity.[15]

The last entry, on October 30, read:

> One hundred and fortieth day. Boyd and Gortz died during night.[16]

Notes

1. G. S. Nares, *Narrative of a Voyage to the Polar Sea During 1875–76 in H.M. Ships Alert and Discovery*, Vol. I and II, 4th ed. (London: Sampson Low, Marston, Searle and Rivington, 1878).

2. A. W. Greely, *Three Years of Arctic Service. An Account of the Lady Franklin Bay Expedition of 1881–84* (London: Richard Bentley and Son, 1886); A. L. Todd, *Abandon* (New York: McGraw-Hill, 1961).

3. R. T. Reuther, "First President of the Explorers' Club—Major General Aldophus Washington Greely," *The Explorers Journal* 72, 1 (1994): 4–9.

4. See Greely, *Three Years of Arctic Service*, and Greely, *The Attainment of the Farthest North*, Vol 1 and 2 (London: Rich and Bentley and Son, 1886).

5. Ibid.

6. Ibid., Vol. 2, 272.

7. Ibid., Vol. 2, 274.

8. Ibid., Vol. 2, 216.

9. Ibid., Vol. 2, 326.

10. Reuther, 6.

11. W. S. Schley, Report on *Greely Expedition. The Greely Arctic Expedition as Fully Narrated by Lt. Greely, USA, and Other Survivors, Commander Schley's Report* (Philadelphia: Barclay and Co., 1884), 25.

12. James Gordon Bennett, in 1871, sent Henry Stanley to Africa to find David Livingston. Bennett, believing he had another chance for a newspaperman's dream, hoped for an exclusive story that would bring his paper a lot of money.

13. E. DeLong, ed., *The Voyage of the "Jeannette,"* Vol. II (Boston: Houghton, Mifflin Co., 1883), 587.

14. G. W. Melville, *In the Lena Delta* (New York: Houghton, Mifflin and Co., 1885).

15. DeLong, 791.

16. DeLong, 800.

9

The Latter-Day Vikings

After a lapse of the better part of a thousand years, two descendents of the Vikings, the Norwegians Roald Amundsen and Dr. Fridtjof Nansen became champions of polar exploration, carrying a Norwegian flag to and through areas where others had not sailed. Their successes resulted from devising methods tailored for the polar areas rather than adapting naval nonpolar procedures. Thus, they supplanted the British naval squadrons and drew upon their previous extensive experience gained in the course of their discoveries.

Although Amundsen and Nansen had different backgrounds, attitudes, ways of life and accomplishments, these two shared an intense internal drive for polar exploration. Nansen was a scholar and a careful planner; Amundsen was also a careful planner, but cool and calculating every move for success. Nansen, an educated writer with a Ph.D. in marine biology, was famous in the end for his world peace efforts after World War I, culminating when he received the 1922 Nobel Peace Prize. Amundsen wrote little until his final South Pole success, producing a report which, although excellent in information and exactness, was neither a popularized version nor a self-promotion. Amundsen looked up to Nansen as his star but went his own way, with the result that the two of them never became close friends. Nevertheless, their lives were intermittently intertwined. Of the many elements that made their ventures so successful, one that stands out is that they recognized the importance of good, nutritious food and how to ensure its availability.

When these latter-day Vikings conquered the polar areas, they were challenging British domination. Nansen started with a land expedition, which the Norwegians knew how to do well, in addition to their many conquests of the sea. Nansen crossed the Greenland ice cap in the summer of 1888,

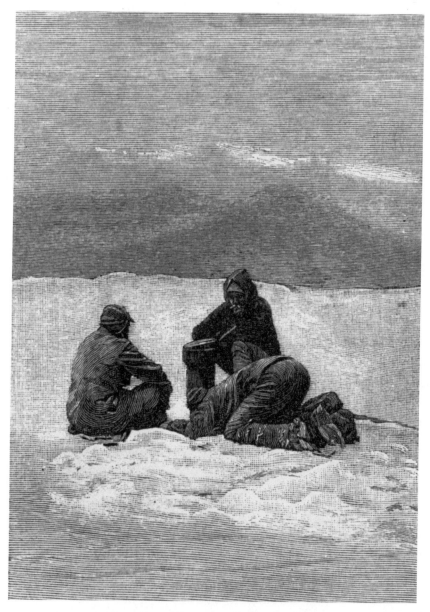

Open air cookery on Nansen's crossing of Greenland. F. Nansen, 1892

accompanied by five companions, including two Norwegian Lapps. The Lapps from northern Norway had desirable knowledge of traveling across snow. This trek also introduced more modern techniques for conquering the poles.

In his fine book, *The First Crossing of Greenland*, Nansen set forth his ideas on transportation, food, and the advantages of traveling with dogs:

> It was my original intention to take, if possible, dogs or reindeer to drag our baggage...At the same time, too, there is this advantage, that one can always procure a supply of fresh meat by slaughtering the animals one by one.
>
> It will no doubt be urged that these advantages will not be gained if dogs are taken. But I can answer from my own experience that hunger is a sufficiently good cook to render dog's flesh anything but unpalatable...If I could obtain good dogs I should therefore have taken them.[1]

He was not able to take dogs on his expedition across the Greenland ice cap, so he made sure that the men could push, pull, or carry all equipment and supplies. Another lesson that he learned for himself and emphasized to others was the importance of fat in the diet on such expeditions. For this trip, he had ordered pemmican from a dealer in Copenhagen but had to make do with simply dried meat, because the dealer failed to prepare the requested product. When the trip was over, he reported that "This was an unpleasant surprise. We suffered from a craving for fat which can scarcely be realized for anyone who does not experience it."[2] Other supplies included a "meat-powder chocolate"—meat powder combined with vegetable fat from a coconut—which he said was "especially useful, as it is both nourishing and palatable."[3] They also carried a preparation of paté from calf liver called "leverpostei," which, they discovered, was totally unsuited to their needs as it contained water which froze and was very difficult to divide: "On ours we broke several knives, and we had eventually to take to the axe; but then it was necessary to go around afterwards to gather up the fragments which flew far and wide over the snow."[4]

Condensed milk and chocolate were a valuable addition. Certainly not inconsequential was Nansen's decision to go from the less populated east coast across to the west coast, which gave them a goal at the end where there was comfort and food.

Five years later another polar adventure began that changed most of the future polar expeditions. This was based on Nansen's theory that the best way to reach the pole was to let a ship drift in the ice pack, and that it might get near enough to the pole to provide a base for attaining that point. This method of reaching the pole was facilitated by the creation of a ship suitable for the conditions. The Scottish designer Colin Archer made the *Fram*, a ship that was built to ride on top of the ice, the first of its kind, so sturdy that it would not be crushed, and if squeezed in the ice, it would pop up. *Fram* was the first truly polar ship.

In the late fall of 1893, with a crew of only twelve, Nansen took the *Fram* into the ice near the New Siberian Islands. His idea, from seeing other things drift in the Arctic, was that there must be a drift around the polar area. The ship was frozen in and eventually was released not far from Spitsbergen; she had drifted almost a quarter of that part of the Arctic. She had even gone near to the pole, as close as perhaps about 300 miles. In preparing for this expedition, food was important: "For the success of such an expedition two things only are required—viz., good clothing and plenty of food, and these we can take care to have with us."[5] As to his foods:

> Special attention was, of course, devoted to our commissariat with a view to obviating the danger of scurvy and other ailments. The principle on which I acted in the choice of provisions was to combine variety with wholesomeness. Every single article of food was chemically analyzed before being adopted, and great care was taken that it should be properly packed. Such articles, even, as bread, dried vegetables, etc. were soldered down in tins as a protection against damp.[6]

Nansen himself left the ship during this time—not because he was concerned about its stability, but because of his interest in reaching the North Pole. He left the *Fram* in March with sledges, dogs, kayaks, skis, and one companion, Hjalmar Johansen, for a dash to the pole. Although they did not make it, they did reach 170 miles farther north than anyone had come before. Even though this alone was enough to make them heroes at home, the return trip was such that Nansen became the polar hero not only of Norway but much of the world.

The two explorers went 500 miles over drifting pack ice, having to kill and eat most of their dogs. They were low in ammunition, and even killed the dogs with knives. They bypassed small prey, such as birds. They rationed their food, which lasted until their first successful killing of a seal. Soon they were intermittently hauling their kayaks and sailing them through leads of ice. Finally they arrived at the Russian islands of Franz Josef Land. Here in August they built a hovel of stones and walrus skins and prepared to spend the winter. With many polar bears and walruses around they had plenty to eat; they suffered no malnutrition, and certainly no scurvy. In May

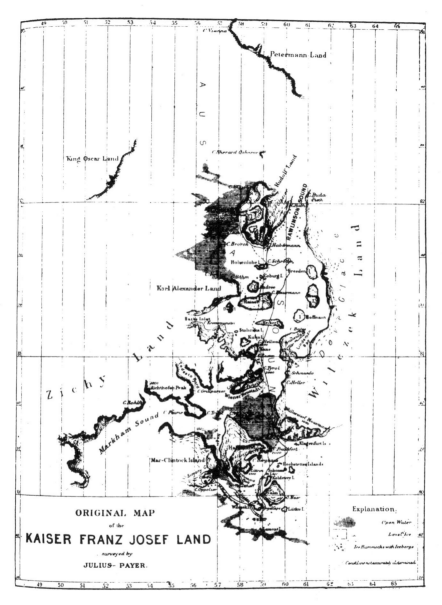

Kaiser Franz Joseph Land. F. Nansen, 1897

of 1896 they headed south, hoping to reach Spitsbergen. Then they had a miraculous encounter with another explorer, Frederick Jackson, and Nansen and Johansen were rescued.

Nansen's success was not just a matter of knowing how to go across the ice and survive, but how to prepare the food.

> The most difficult, but also, perhaps, the most important, point in the equipment of a sledge expedition is thoroughly good and adequate victualling....[T]he first and foremost object is to protect one's self against scurvy and other maladies by the choice of foods, which, through careful preparation and sterilization, are assured against decomposition. On a sledge expedition of this kind, where so much attention must be paid to the weight of the equipment, it is hardly possible to take any kinds of provisions except those of which the weight has been reduced as much as possible by careful and complete drying. As, however, meat and fish are not so easily digested when dried, it is no unimportant thing to have them in a pulverized form. The dried food is, in this manner, so finely distributed that it can with equal facility be digested and received into the organism. This preparation of meat and fish was, therefore, the only kind we took with us. The meat was muscular beef, taken from the ox, and freed from all fat, gristle, etc.; it was then dried as quickly as possible, in a completely fresh condition, and thereupon ground and mixed with the same proportion of beef suet as is used in the ordinary preparation of pemmican. This form of food, which has been used for a considerable time on sledge expeditions, has gained for itself much esteem, and rightly; if well prepared, as ours was, it is undeniably a nourishing and easily digested food. I had also had prepared a large quantity of pemmican, consisting of equal parts of meat-powder and vegetable fat (from the coconut). This pemmican, however, proved to be rather an unfortunate invention; even the dogs would not eat it after they had tasted it once or twice. Perhaps this is accounted for by the fact that vegetable fat is not easily digested, and contains acids which irritate the mucous membranes of the stomach and throat. One ought not, however, to trust to its always being harmless, as, if carelessly prepared—i.e., slowly or imperfectly dried—it may also be very injurious to the health.
>
> Another item of our provisions, by which we set great store, was Vage's fish-flour. It is well prepared and has admirable keeping qualities; if boiled in water and mixed with flour and butter or dried potatoes, it furnishes a very appetizing dish. Another point which should be attended to is that the food be of such a kind that it can be eaten without cooking. Fuel is part of an equipment, no doubt; but if for some reason or other this be lost or used up, one would be in a bad case indeed had one not provided against such a contingency by taking food which could be eaten in spite of that. In order to save fuel, too, it is important that the food should not require cooking, but merely warming. The flour that we took with us had therefore been steamed, and could, if necessary, have been eaten as it was, without further preparation. Merely brought to a boil, it made a good hot dish. We also took dried boiled potatoes, pea-soup, chocolate, vril-food , etc. Our bread was partly carefully dried wheaten biscuits, and partly aleuronate bread, which

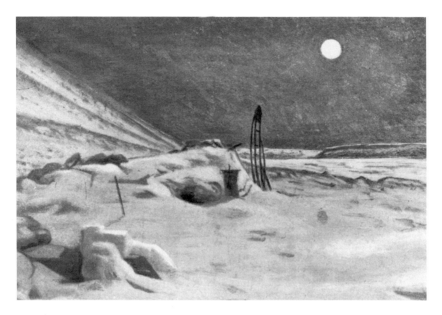

Nansen's winter hut. F. Nansen, 1897

I had caused to be made of wheat flour mixed with about 30 per cent of aleuronate flour (vegetable albumen).

We also took with us a considerable quantity of butter (86 pounds) which had been well worked on board in order to get out all superfluous water. By this means not only was considerable weight saved, but the butter did not become so hard in the cold. On the whole, it must be said that our menus included considerable variety, and we were never subjected to that sameness of food which former sledge expeditions have complained so much of. Finally, we always had ravenous appetites, and always thought our meals as delicious as they could be.[7]

Water was also a necessity that Nansen understood very well and he knew how to obtain it:

For melting water in the cooker it is better to use ice than snow, particularly if the latter be not old and granular. Newly fallen snow gives little water, and requires considerably more heat to warm it. That part of salt-water ice which is above the surface of the sea, and, in particular, prominent pieces which have been exposed to the rays of the sun during a summer and are thus freed from the greater part of their salt, furnish excellent drinking water. Some expeditions have harbored the superstition that drinking-water from ice in which there was the least salt was injurious. This is a mistake which cost, for instance, the members of the *Jeannette* expedition much unnecessary trouble, as they thought it imperative to distil the water before they could drink it without incurring the risk of scurvy.[8]

Nansen, the explorer, scientist, politician, and Nobel Peace Prize winner, was also a first-class practical nutritionist. His observations on polar operations, Eskimos, and rations set a standard for Amundsen, Peary, Cook, and others for the next two decades.

The other latter-day Viking, Roald Amundsen, became enamored with polar travel as a young teenager, primarily as an ardent admirer of Nansen. From then on he devoted his life to polar struggles. Shipping out early to the southern hemisphere and then soon afterwards on northern whalers, he earned his seaman's papers. With his master's papers, he even went to Antarctica on a Belgian ship, the *Belgica*, where he became a close friend of another northern polar explorer, Dr. Frederick Cook. On the *Belgica* voyage, Amundsen had a serious bout of scurvy towards the end of the winter, and Cook's earlier poorly received entreaties to the captain to lay up penguin meat for health sank deeply into Amundsen's mind.[9]

Cook, in turn, had become a seasoned polar explorer from an expedition in the Arctic with Robert Peary. Cook described what could have been a major disaster, but what became only a minor incident because of what Cook called Amundsen's "presence of mind":

> April 4 (1898): There has been a great excitement today one which has forced a new interest into the sameness of the daily routine (on shipboard, frozen into the ice). The woodwork about the pipe of the cabin stove became ignited, and for a few seconds there was a cry of fire and a great scramble for water. Amundsen, with admirable presence of mind, drew out the pipe from the deck and then smothered the flames with snow, while the rest of us hustled for water, which is always scarce on the *Belgica*.[10]

From the *Belgica* experiences and teachings of Cook, Amundsen soon matured into a leader and an accomplished polar explorer. He completed his later voyages in the Arctic and his trip to the South Pole without an incident of scurvy.

Amundsen was renowned for his first attainment of the South Pole. Equally significant, perhaps, in the eyes of polar ship captains, was his discovery of the northwest passage, a prize the pursuit of which had resulted in the deaths of many men and caused many ships to founder. With but little financial help and going into serious debt, he outfitted a ship called the *Gjoa*, which was but seventy-five feet long and more than thirty years old. It had been a fishing boat and was, indeed, a poor vessel for conquering the Arctic. In early June of 1902 he left Norway with a crew of seven. He took seven not only because the ship was small but also because he knew, from his extensive studies and acquired knowledge, that a small complement had a better chance of surviving in areas where the acquisition of food from the environment might mean the difference between life and death. He knew that Nansen had made it across miles of ice in Greenland with only three, and in the polar sea with only two. He also knew that larger expeditions had experienced starvation.

Amundson and his crew succeeded in crossing the Atlantic, and though they experienced many small problems, they were able to surmount them all. He even received help from Eskimos on reaching Greenland. On August 22 they reached Beechey Island and anchored briefly in Erebus Bay. They left Erebus Bay to anchor by King William Land in an area which they called Gjoa Haven. Here they stayed for nearly two years. With his background in polar exploration, both in the north and in the south with Cook, Amundsen knew how important it was to supplement their diet with fresh meat, and an opportunity to do so presented itself. The area where he and the crew anchored was along an established route of migration for caribou. It took only a few weeks for the men to acquire enough meat and freeze it in the arctic frost to last them all winter.

During this time at Gjoa Haven, they made many important side explorations. They lived and worked with Eskimos, continuously learning the skills of survival. When Amundsen found that their limited number of dogs did not haul the loads well for an exploring group of four men, he immediately changed the number of men to two but kept the same number of dogs. There were no problems with illness because the group was small, and with the Eskimo teachings they were able to live off the land, just as Amundsen had planned—again a victory for detailed planning. They were able to sail forth on August 13, 1905, and on August 27 they completed the northwest passage, where they were met by an American ship coming around from the northern tip of Alaska—and all this without a single case of scurvy or malnutrition.[11]

Notes

1. F. Nansen, *The First Crossing of Greenland* (London: Longmans, Green and Co., 1892), 21.
2. Ibid., 39.
3. Ibid.
4. Ibid.
5. F. Nansen, *Farthest North* (New York: Harper and Brothers, 1898), 45.
6. Ibid.
7. Ibid., 362.

8. Ibid., 419.

9. F. A. Cook, *Through the First Antarctic Night* (New York: Doubleday and McClure Co, 1900), 246.

10. Ibid., 234, 236. Fires for cooking and heating are dangerous in polar areas because they can easily spread from the winds, and there is usually no water at hand, only ice and sometimes ice-like snow.

11. R. Amundsen, *The Northwest Passage* (London: A. Constable and Co., 1908).

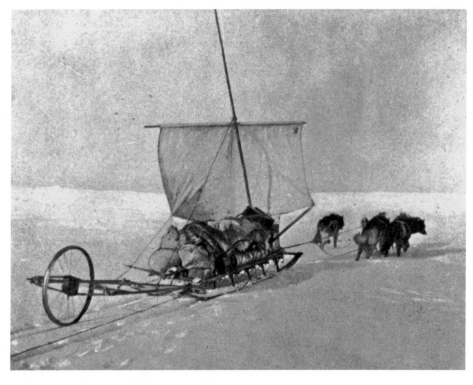

Peary sailing over the inland ice. J. D. Peary, 1894

10

Races to the North Pole: Robert Peary and Frederick Cook

During the first decade of the 20th century two individuals, Robert Edwin Peary and Dr. Frederick Cook, both claimed to have reached the North Pole. Peary's claim was accepted initially, while Cook's was repudiated except by a few. These were two extraordinarily different men.

Peary was born in 1856, spent his youth in Maine, and graduated from Bowdoin College in civil engineering. After he was commissioned in the U.S. Navy, he worked on plans for a canal across Nicaragua. However, he soon became consumed by arctic exploration, possibly from reading the thrilling writings of Kane and others; it was to be a lifelong passion. Peary was a career arctic explorer, with a long-time dedication to conquering the pole during his many arctic trips. He had learned the procedures and habits of Eskimos, including the use of dogs, and he communicated closely with the Eskimos, as well as including them in his support teams.

In 1886 he went on his first exploration during a summer in Greenland, and it was enough to change his life. In 1891 he sailed with his wife, Elvin de Astrup, of Norway, Matthew Henson, the first African-American among famous northern names, and Dr. Frederick Cook, who served as a volunteer doctor.[1] Peary claimed the discovery of new areas and was extensively acclaimed. In 1893, he again went with his wife and a supporter of his, Harry Bartlet, to Whale Sound. Trying to go north he was stopped by sea ice and had to turn back. In 1894 Bartlet returned to the ship and took the group back to Philadelphia except Peary, Henson, and the Eskimo Hug Lee. The three of them, plus six other Eskimos and sixty dogs, tried a northeast route toward the pole. This was nearly a complete disaster, and they almost lost their lives on being storm-bound and struggling over disintegrating ice. But Peary learned from the experience.[2]

Over the years, Peary became the most traveled and most knowledgeable of polar explorers regarding ice and snow travel. He always went with, and lived with, Eskimos, learned their ways, and adopted many of their techniques. (South polar explorers did not have the advantage of Eskimo companions, although these explorers could have profited—and a very few did—from knowledge of Eskimo techniques.) In contrast to many explorers still to follow, Peary did not carry tents in winter travels, but rather made igloos; he did not carry a sleeping bag, but rather wore it, his hooded parka and Eskimo-style pants. Some points in the so-called "Peary System," as he summarized his procedures, were:

> To drive a ship through the ice to the farthest possible northern land base from which she can be driven back again the following year.
>
> To do enough hunting during the fall and winter to keep the party healthily supplied with fresh meat.
>
> To have dogs enough to allow for the loss of sixty per cent of them by death or otherwise.
>
> To have the confidence of a large number of Eskimos, earned by square dealing and generous gifts in the past, so that they will follow the leader to any point he may specify.
>
> To transport beforehand to the point where the expedition leaves the land for the sledge journey, sufficient food, fuel, clothing, stoves (oil or alcohol) and other mechanical equipment to get the main party to the Pole and back and the various divisions to their farthest north and back.
>
> To have every item of equipment of the quality best suited to the purpose, thoroughly tested, and of the lightest possible weight.
>
> To return by the same route followed on the upward march, using the beaten trail and the already constructed igloos to save the time and strength that would have been expended in constructing new igloos and in trail-breaking.
>
> To know exactly to what extent each man and dog may be worked without injury.
>
> Last, but not least, to have the absolute confidence of every member of the party, white, black, or brown, so that every order of the leader will be implicitly obeyed.[3]

It is worth noting among these thoughtful if Victorian-sounding points, the pride of place given to the importance of food ("to keep the party healthily supplied with fresh meat") in both quality and quantity ("for the sledge journey, sufficient food...").

Peary's avowed successful trip to the North Pole began in 1908 when he sailed in the spring with two good ships and with very expensive privately

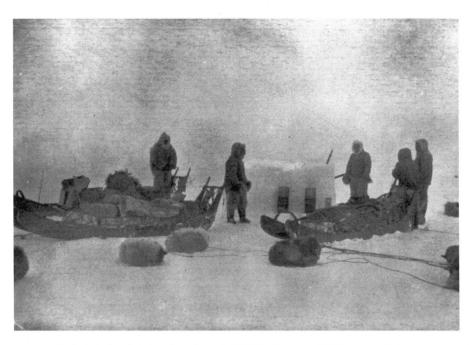

The halt for lunch in last forced march (89° 25 minutes to 89° 57 minutes), showing alcohol stores in snow shelter. R. E. Peary, 1910

donated provisions and equipment for his exploration.[4] He even had a send-off from President Teddy Roosevelt. On his way north he stopped at a place where Dr. Frederick Cook claimed he had left much of his materials and records for reaching the pole. (Cook claimed that Peary made off with Cook's records. There is a very strong question about what really happened at this place.) Peary continued on the ship with 260 dogs and fifty Eskimos and put out food and fuel depots on land to the north. In the middle of February he sent teams forth toward the pole, with Peary himself soon following. This was a big expedition, with nearly thirty sledges and 140 dogs. Starting at 87°47 minutes latitude, Peary went on with Henson and three Eskimos to the pole. Starting back on April 7, they reached the ship by the 25th. His speed was so great that some still doubt that he had reached the pole, but at that time the doubters were very few, and Peary was acclaimed as the "discoverer of the North Pole."[5]

The other claimant for reaching the North Pole, Dr. Frederick Cook, was born in 1865, and educated in New York at the College of Physicians and Surgeons. Cook was a dreamer and a loner who possessed a love of

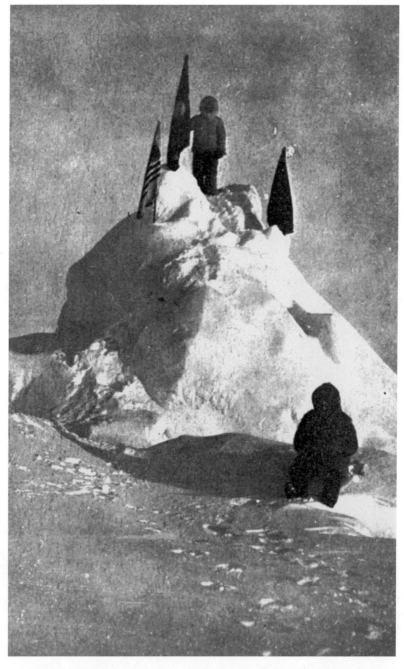

Peary's photograph of the stars and stripes flying at the North Pole. R. E. Peary, 1917

adventure. Nearly ten years younger than Peary, he was just a few years behind him in going to the Arctic.

As is often found, purposeful men with similar interests and objectives can become enemies as well as competitors; so it was with Peary and Cook. Cook had been sent to visit Peary's rear base in 1901 at a time when Peary's backers were concerned about disease at the encampment.[6] When Cook saw that Peary had lost most of his toes on both feet from frostbite, he told Peary that his polar explorations were finished. From this and other happenings, the two were never friends again. Cook then formed a close association with another polar explorer, Roald Amundsen. The two men had met in 1898 on Adrien de Gerlache's ship, the *Belgica*, that went to Antarctica.[7]

With his arctic training behind him and after his antarctic experience, Cook was ready to attack the North Pole.[8] In July 1907 he left New York with little fanfare and certainly no ostentatious good-bye parties. His expedition was financed by only one person, sportsman John R. Bradley. He sailed to Annoatok, the northernmost settlement on the globe, where he made a decision to dash for the pole. An advance party with Eskimos and dogs, all of which he arranged while there, laid out some supplies towards the pole. Near the end of February 1908 Cook broke off from the advance party and went towards the pole with two Eskimos.

According to Cook, they started with twenty-six dogs and a boat, the latter, which Peary did not have, enabling them to cross water. The story of his trip to the North Pole is a gripping one. With limited equipment they lived off the land much of the way, but even so they were short of rations upon reaching the pole on April 21, 1908.

The story of the trip back is one that should make every young person yearn to try.[9] With dogs gone, supplies very low, and finally reduced to no ammunition, they had to learn how to spear and trap animals for food. Death seemed imminent several times. It is not known why all the trouble occurred when Cook knew so much about the north and polar living, although two outstanding reasons could be the very small size of his support group and the fact that he lost his way for part of the trip.

Cook's description of the importance of the boat and his attitude towards food and nutrition show his understanding of their critical roles:

> We found such a canoe boat to fit the situation exactly, and selected a twelve-foot boat with wooden frame. The slats, spreaders and floor-pieces were utilized as parts of sledges. The canvas cover served as a floor cloth for our sleeping bags. Thus the boat did useful service for a hundred days and never

seemed needlessly cumbersome. When the craft was finally spread for use as a boat, in it we carried the sledge, in it we sought game for food, and in it or under it we camped. Without it we could never have returned.

Even more vital than the choice of sledges, more vital than anything else, I knew, in such a trip as I proposed, is the care of the stomach. From the published accounts of Arctic traveling it is impossible to learn a fitting ration, and I hasten to add that I well realized that our own experience may not solve the problem for future expeditions. The gastronomic need differs with every man. It differs with every expedition, and it is radically different with every nation. Thus, when de Gerlache, with good intentions, forced Norwegian food into French stomachs, he learned that there is a nationality in gastronomics. Nor is it safe to listen to scientific advice, for the stomach is arbitrary, and stands as autocrat over every human sense and passion and will not easily yield to dictates.

In this respect, as in others, I was helped very much by the natives. The Eskimo is ever hungry, but his taste is normal. Things of doubtful value in nutrition form no part in his diet. Animal food, consisting of meat and fat, is entirely satisfactory as a steady diet without other adjuncts. His food requires neither salt nor sugar, nor is cooking a matter of necessity.

Quantity is important, but quality applies only to the relative proportion of fat. With this key to gastronomics, pemmican was selected as the staple food, and it would also serve equally well for the dogs.

We had an ample supply of pemmican, which was made of pounded dried beef, sprinkled with a few raisins and some currants, and slightly sweetened with sugar. This mixture was cemented together with heated beef tallow and run into tin cans containing six pounds each.

This combination was invented by the American Indian, and the supply for this expedition was made by Armour of Chicago after a formula furnished by Captain Evelyn B. Baldwin. Pemmican had been used before as part of the long list of foodstuffs for Arctic expeditions, but with us there was the important difference that it was to be almost entirely the whole bill of fare when away from game haunts. The palate surprises in our store were few.[10]

A still-unsolved dispute exists over whether Cook really made it to the pole, and if evidence and supplies cached at a station in the Arctic were molested by Peary on his later return. If Cook's claim had held, he would have been first to reach the North Pole, but eventually his claim was discredited by much of the world. Added to this was a strongly supported assertion that Cook's previous climb of Mt. McKinley in Alaska was a hoax.[11] The establishment recognized him for nothing. A very, very sad end came later when Cook, convicted in 1923 of fraud by the government on oil lands, was sent to Leavenworth prison. Although pardoned in 1940 by Franklin Delano Roosevelt, he had remained in prison until 1930. This pardon did not come soon enough, because Cook died a few months later.[12]

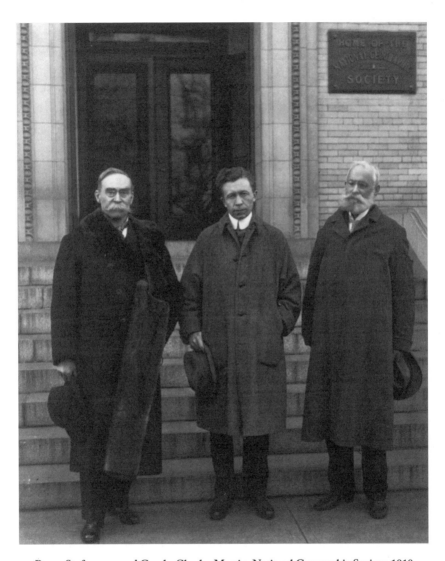

Peary, Stefansson, and Greely. Charles Martin, National Geographic Society, 1919

Robert Peary was ambitious, hard-driving, tough, and an expert polar explorer who generally found success with his numerous well-planned, well-executed polar trips. Frederick Cook was an extra-establishment dreamer and adventurer. Peary was the confidant and mentor to many polar explorers, Cook the coexplorer with two of the great names of polar success—with Peary himself and with Amundsen. Planning, administrating, and executing, as done by Peary, usually made for success. Current thought is that Peary possibly could have stopped about 100 miles from the pole because his time of travel was too short for the distance claimed. Considering Peary's many fine arctic explorations, his tenacity, and his perseverance, however, one might believe that he deserved credit for reaching the pole.

Regardless of the questions concerning the authenticity of Cook's North Pole venture, his books have vivid descriptions of a man fighting for his life and yet conquering polar living. Although some, like Amundsen and others, gave him credit for finding the pole and regarded him as a hero, still others thought he was a charlatan, and a few considered him to be an outright liar.[13] Berton quotes Peter Freuchen as thinking Cook a liar but also a gentleman,[14] and Peary was neither. Worse, Stefansson, on questioning Eskimos, was told that Cook did not have a shortage of ammunition, in fact even encouraged target practice.[15] Was a shortage of ammunition a valid reason for his miraculous tale of hunting with prehistoric weapons for food? Perhaps Peary did not make the exact pole because of lack of food. Perhaps Cook had plenty of food. In an attempt to solve finally Peary's claim, the National Geographic Society commissioned a reexamination of Peary's photographs by photogrammetric rectification, a technique based on shadows.[16] His position was calculated to have been where he had claimed to be. Even so, the arguments continue.

Notes

1. J. D. Peary, *My Antarctic Journal: A Year Among the Ice Fields and Eskimoes* (New York: Contemporary Publ. Co., 1894).
2. R. E. Peary, *Northward Over the Great Ice,* Vol. 2 (New York: F. A. Stokes, 1898), 148–152.
3. R. E. Peary, *The North Pole* (New York: F. A. Stokes, 1910), 202.
4. Ibid., 4.
5. Ibid., 363.
6. P. Berton, *The Arctic Grail* (New York: Viking Penguin, 1988), 528.
7. F. A. Cook, *Through the First Antarctic Night* (New York: Doubleday and McClure, 1900), xi.

8. F. A. Cook, *My Attainment of the Pole* (New York: Lent and Griff, 1911), 23.

9. F. A. Cook, *Return from the Pole* (New York: Pellegrini and Cudahy, 1951), 58.

10. Cook, *My Attainment of the Pole,* 134.

11. D. Rawlins, *Peary at the North Pole. Fact or Fiction?* (Washington: Robert B. Luce, 1973), 135.

12. H. S. Abraham, *Hero in Disgrace* (New York: Paragon House, 1971), 210.

13. W. R. Hunt, *To Stand at the Pole* (New York: Stein and Day, 1981), 256.

14. Berton, *The Arctic Grail,* 623.

15. Cook, *Return from the Pole,* 234–236.

16. T. D. Davies, "New Evidence Places Peary at the Pole," *National Geographic* 177, 1 (1990): 44.

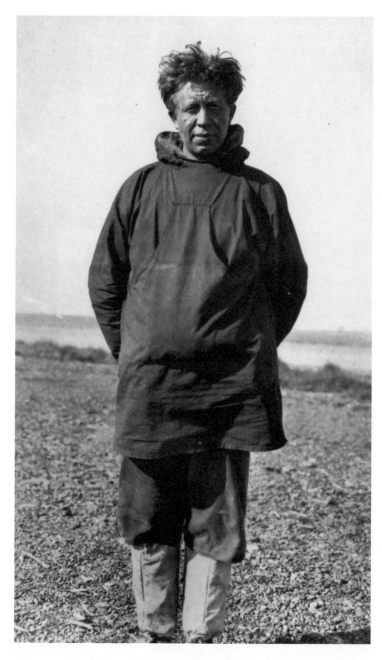

Vilhjalmur Stefansson. Alaska and Polar Regions Department, Rasmuson Library, University of Alaska Fairbanks

11

The Almost Eskimo:
Vilhjalmur Stefansson

Vilhjalmur Stefansson was considered by many to be the "almost Eskimo," because he embraced the lifestyle of the Native people with whom he was closely associated during his travels. Stefansson was a scholar, writer, adventurer, promoter, anthropologist, sociologist, and nutritionist—something like a human melting pot. Nancy Fogelson has described him as Canada's counterpart to Peary.[1] Perhaps it was this all-encompassing mix that has made specialists in different fields question some of his work, some of his findings, and many of his interpretations and recommendations.

A prolific writer, he published some twenty books, gave many lectures, and engaged in actual experimentation. Living like an Eskimo, Stefansson even tried to think like an Eskimo. From his study of the Eskimo diet he showed how a few individuals could live in most areas of the Arctic, more or less off the land. He soon developed a consuming drive for recommending the value of an all-meat diet. Of his many books, three are sufficiently different to give a general flavor of him in history: *The Friendly Arctic* (1921), *Hunters of the Great North* (1944), and *Not by Bread Alone* (1946).[2]

Stefansson came from a pioneer family that first settled in the woods of Manitoba, Canada, in 1876.[3] While there, the family apparently lost a brother and sister to malnutrition. Vilhjalmur was born in 1879; he moved to a farm in North Dakota when he was less than two years old. There he grew up and, after his father's death, came close to becoming a cowboy. With only fifty-three dollars for his education, he left home to work his way through college. He attended the University of North Dakota, but less than a year from graduation left the university. He was probably one of the brightest students there. Somehow he managed to go to the University of Iowa, where a year later, in 1903 at the age of twenty-three, he graduated. Then he was on to Harvard, where he began his study of anthropology. In 1906, as a result of some of his writings on Greenland colonies, Stefansson was offered the possibility to go on an expedition studying Eskimos.

Stefansson's major arctic explorations were divided into three separate ventures, all dealing with his deep interest in Eskimo anthropology and arctic nutrition. The first—sometimes called the Leffingwell-Mikkelson expedition—was in 1906–1907, while he was still studying at Harvard, and made possible with financial assistance from both Harvard University and the University of Toronto. The second exploration lasted four years from 1908–1912 and was sponsored by the American Museum of Natural History and the Geological Survey of Canada. The third was a five-year one, 1913–1918, entirely sponsored by the Canadian government.

When he was offered his first chance in 1906, he immediately accepted and planned to meet the expedition members at their forward base on Herschel Island the next spring. After reaching the island he was met by the captain of a whaling ship who told him that the ship bringing the exploring group had met with some problems in the ice and the complement would not arrive for another year. Turning down an invitation from the captain to sail back to Point Barrow, Stefansson stayed on Herschel Island and lived a whole year with the Eskimos, learning their customs and their language and eating their food. He was meeting the Arctic on its own terms. On returning to the United States in 1907, he decided to launch his own expedition (his second) in order to study a tribe of Eskimos who lived far north, some of whom reputedly had light skin and light hair. When Stefansson was in the Arctic, some setbacks delayed his expedition for two years. He finally started off with two Eskimos, a sled and a team of dogs for Cape Parry, where supposedly the light-haired Eskimos lived. On Victoria Island he reported tall, blue-eyed Eskimos, with every appearance of perhaps being descended from white explorers. Apparently isolated for some time, their culture was more that of the stone age than was that of other Eskimo tribes further south. Their true origin has never been established.

For two more years Stefansson quietly continued his studies. He was quite well known when he returned to the United States, and it was then that he propounded that the most important point of his work was showing how people could live off the land and on the Eskimo diet. On a diet of caribou, fish, and seal, one might get a little bit bored, but it served the purpose well.

His next objective was to show that man could find enough game on the central ice pack to live away from land. To do this, he planned his third expedition for 1913–1918. This included a 500-mile trip across the ice with only two companions and without any provisions. He obtained $150,000 backing from the Canadian government, which had more than just an interest in anthropology. Much of the arctic north of Canada needed more attention to support Canada's claim for sovereignty. So, even with the war in Europe, Stefansson had both governmental and financial support for his anthropology research and his interest in nutrition. All went well when he set off for the ice, but there was a catastrophe from loss of the expedition's vessel, the *Karluk*, before he started wherein much of the equipment was destroyed and eight men were lost. On March 22, 1914, he headed off with two well-seasoned Norwegian explorers. Two months later they were out on the ice and food was low. But after Stefansson shot a polar bear that had attacked him, they had the food they needed for themselves and the dogs and had proven his belief that food was there.

The third exploration had been divided into two, Stefansson's northern party and another southern party, headed by the Canadian naturalist Rudolph M. Anderson, Stefansson's coexplorer during his second exploration. Well qualified as an explorer and a naturalist, Anderson led a very successful and extensive study in several fields, including mineralogy and geology, both of intense interest to the Canadian government. Problems related to food did not occur, and he was acclaimed for his excellent work.

Anderson's relationship with Stefansson soured, however, and Anderson later described Stefansson merely as a "clever writer and talker."[4] Much of this arose from an opinion of Anderson and others that Stefansson had abandoned the *Karluk*, leaving it to its fateful sinking and the death of members of the team. To give another side of the argument, perhaps Stefansson had wanted to train them in survival, but they had refused it.

Stefansson went on more visits to the Arctic, with many exploits. At all times he observed, studied, noted, and eventually reported. Although he supplied dramatic descriptions of the land and its wildlife, some of his critics have thought his knowledge of ecology was defective. Barry Lopez, whose own accounts of the Arctic are notable, wrote that Stefansson's knowledge of arctic biology was flawed and that he wanted to make nature over to suit his own beliefs.[5] Stefansson believed, for example, that the vegetation was wasted on caribou and should be replaced by cattle. Apparently he did not consider how the vegetation would be affected or the problems of survival for cattle in an arctic environment.

Still, Stefansson revered the Arctic and its people and understood its dangers. In contrast to descriptions of the north as a barren, silent, and frozen place,[6] Stefansson and his companions found it hospitable and friendly. It was easier to stay warm by wearing proper clothing than to remain comfortable in extremely warm temperatures. Though people might freeze to death in the north, the cause was usually accident or carelessness. Living in warm climates was not without risk; consider sunstroke. Thus, living in the far north suited Stefansson just fine, though he believed it was an individual's responsibility to adjust to it.

On Stefansson's first arctic trip, when he found himself to be without his expedition party for a year, he not only lived with the Eskimos he initially encountered, but he also traveled with them when they visited other tribes. He sought those who were reported to be less sophisticated because they had not been as closely involved with the white sealers and explorers. He started his journey at a place called Shingle Point on Herschel Island near the Mackenzie Delta. Soon he encountered extraordinary company when Amundsen's ship, the *Gjoa*, with Amundsen aboard, stopped on the concluding leg of his famous passage across the Arctic. With advice from Amundsen and others Stefansson decided to move. He left for a small Eskimo town where he lived long enough to learn their language, their customs, and how to live off the land. Stefansson soon overcame his childhood dislike of fish and became a complete fish eater—without salt or tea or anything else—as this was the only thing available to eat.[7] For awhile, he ate only the best fish specially prepared for him. It was not long, however, before he joined the Eskimos and ate right from their potfuls of boiled mixed fish parts. Fish heads were a different problem, requiring several months before he agreed with the Eskimos' opinions that fish heads were the best parts of the fish—in their opinion, a real delicacy. The same applied to caribou heads, and Stefansson came to believe that people who ate an exclusively meat diet all had this preference for heads—not only Eskimos and Indians, but also white men.

In Stefansson's many books are descriptions of the food and diets of Eskimos from the different regions of the Arctic. He frequently included information about their fears and taboos related to food. Of particular interest to modern toxicologists and nutritionists were his on-the-spot investigations of the possible toxicity of seal and polar bear liver, now known to be caused by the enormous excess of vitamin A stored in these mammals' organs. He wrote a lengthy summation of the symptoms he and his colleagues had on eating livers, either purposely as a test or incidentally as part of their diets. At one meal, four of them ate bear liver. Although two of the four became very ill, they were all well by the following day.[8] Two other members of his party were at a different camp and both suffered greatly from eating bear liver. Like the two with Stefansson, they developed violent headaches and nausea, and weakness continued for two more days.

All of this led him to run an experiment. One night his party of four divided up a bear liver and consumed it at about 10:00 P.M. At about four in the morning one colleague was very nauseated and had violent headaches, but Stefansson himself only had a loss of appetite. Members of his party refused to eat bear liver ever again after the experiment, but Stefansson continued to eat it sometimes, though he apparently preferred other meat.

Like most all polar explorers, Stefansson continued his interest in polar explorations until the time of his death at nearly eighty years of age. In contrast to most polar explorers, he spent over half his life, and especially the last thirty years, fighting for his belief in the nutritional value of an Eskimo diet: the consumption of large amounts of meats and fish. He was examined carefully by medical doctors and clinics and in all cases was found to be in excellent health. After nearly a decade of discussions and negotiations, in 1928–1929 Stefansson arranged for the Russell Sage Institute of Pathology to conduct extensive experiments, known as the Cornell-Bellevue Tests, to test his theory that an all-meat diet was not only safe but healthy.[9] So many arguments ensued as to how the experiments should be run that Stefansson had to go to great lengths to ensure that there were no possible loopholes or weak links that critics could later use to condemn and destroy the results of the experiments.[10]

Vegetarians, dieticians, and scientists proved to be the most formidable opponents. The opponents' concerns were based in part on the fact that very high-fat diets under some conditions were known to cause ketosis (the accumulation of oxidation products and acidosis), and it was generally believed then that the energy from carbohydrates helps utilization of fats. High-protein diets could cause kidney damage. Opponents also suspected that scurvy would develop.[11]

Stefansson and a member of his third expedition, Karsten Andersen, were the subjects of the experiment.[12] When the two entered the dietetic ward of Bellevue Hospital, Stefansson reported that strong protests arose over their food and eating habits after a rumor was started that they were going to eat only lean, raw meat. Other issues had to be addressed such as providing supervision of meals at restaurants. During the experiment, the two men were also allowed to attend dinner parties, but Stefansson discussed possible menus with the hostess in advance to ensure that suitable dishes were served. Then, debate arose, particularly in the press, over what constituted an all-meat diet. Opinions differed, for example, over whether to include eggs, milk, and cheese in an all-meat diet. Since some believed they were compatible with a vegetarian's diet, all dairy products and eggs were excluded. Throughout the experiment, Andersen and Stefansson received regular medical tests. This included numerous spells in calorimeters, blood pressure checks, and colon examinations, as well as other general physical notations on their general health.

When the experiment ended, Stefansson concluded it was a rousing victory for his all-meat diet. Though the transition from Andersen's well-balanced and varied diet to an all-meat diet resulted in some minor digestive and colonic problems, he had adjusted to an all-meat diet in a matter of weeks without incident. Indeed, the two men thought that they were in better than average health. They did as well in midsummer as in midwinter, with no more discomfort from the heat than other fellow New Yorkers. Since they were relatively low in carbohydrates during the tests, special examinations for glucose tolerance were done at the conclusion of the experiment. The men were given large quantities in the first test which showed that when they were at first off the meat diet they had a poor sugar tolerance; but "in a week or so we were back to where we had been before the meat year began." During the experiment Stefansson averaged about 2,600 calories a day, with 2,100 from fat, 500 from protein, and with carbohydrates contributing less than 50 calories. There was no deterioration of teeth and a notable absence of pyorrhea. As to their bowels, the stools were nonodorous and there was no evidence of gaseous distention from flatus at any time. As to weight, Stefansson's original weight was 72.5 kilograms, 68 kilograms at the end of the first month, and 69.4 kilograms at the end of the year. Possibly of particular importance in today's medical considerations, this diet did not appear to have any ill-effect on the kidneys.

Stefansson lived a long life, with only the usual illnesses that accompanied the aging of a man at that time. At seventy he began to suffer from arthritis, first in his knee and then in his shoulders. On his seventy-fifth birthday he was going strong, despite a mild stroke that he suffered the year before. The illness of U.S. President Dwight Eisenhower brought public attention to the connection between ill health and eating too much animal fat. Given his own experience, however, Stefansson was not dissuaded from his belief that an all-meat, high-fat diet was healthy. He even recommended including eggs and butter in the diet. By his seventy-sixth birthday he was still doing fine and claimed that even his stiff joints were not as stiff.

In addition to his belief that an all-meat diet was nutritionally sound, at the start of World War II Stefansson campaigned vigorously and vociferously as well for the inclusion of pemmican as a major constituent of military rations for the Armed Forces. Stefansson's biggest defeat probably was in his failure to get the military to agree with him and to adopt pemmican as a special ration during World War II. In *Not By Bread Alone*, following his descriptions of actual shootings between suppliers of pemmican in southern Canada in the 19th century, which he termed the First Pemmican War, he named this battle with the military the Second Pemmican War. The first war was the effort to control the supply of pemmican, and thus the supply routes for obtaining the rich animal pelts in Canada, while the second one was over beliefs regarding the adequacy and wholesomeness of pemmican. Stefansson believed that the Second Pemmican War may have cost lives by denying troops in planes and at the front the best emergency rations.[13] Although there were no massacres, the emotions, politics, and verbal accusations were so intense he felt justified in calling it a war. Stefansson's feelings also ran high.

There were several sides to the arguments. Stefansson believed that the feeling against pemmican went way back to the early times of the settlers of the American continent. He thought that the earliest users of pemmican were trappers and settlers who, in forging forward, had learned the value of the Indian diet. But as families came, and particularly as the women of the households were involved, there was an effort to maintain a tie with their own customs and particularly to be more civilized. Consequently, items like pemmican, strictly Indian food in their opinion, were omitted. This attitude, Stefansson believed, held all the way through to the time of World War II. Pemmican, considered Indian food, was thought of as an unscientifically developed food and consequently something that should not be used in such a highly technical war as the Second World War. Stefansson more or less refused to admit that the science of that time could improve on such more "relatively ancient" foods. His battle, consequently, was not only with dietary custom but with the scientists, including both the analytical chemists and the dieticians, as well as the medical community at large.

Another problem in all these discussions was the definition of pemmican. Almost all of the original pemmican used by explorers was made from lean meat and selected animal fat. Sometimes a few items like berries were included to give variation. However, as pemmican was used and developed with time, other additives were made, and these not only changed the nutritional value of the pemmican but also greatly influenced its keeping qualities. These changes were almost without exception negative ones. Stefansson wrote, "'The modern' pemmicans that contained ground up bacon, shredded coconut, butter, pea meal and the like spoil quickly. They cannot be used on long summer journeys unless canned." Stefansson was further insulted when the navy gave the name pemmican to a candy bar that contained not only a great deal of sugar, vegetable oil and peanuts but even added chocolate to take the place of lean beef—and then "to get a ruling passed by the Navy on the basis of this candy mixture that pemmican should not be used because it is thirst provoking!" Finally, almost entirely due to Stefansson's efforts, the military made some field tests, but these limited tests, done under conditions where the mens' lives were not dependent upon the food, did not prove the value of pemmican.[14]

Pemmican's value, however, was shown much later by the 1986 Steger International Polar Expedition.[15] In retracing Peary's route to the pole, seven men and one woman made the trip with forty-nine sled dogs. Although it was only to the pole and not back, the trip was fifty-five days long, and pemmican was a major item in their diet. During the expedition, their mean energy intake was 7812 Kcals per day with 65.7% of the energy from fat. At the end, although their mean cholesterol values were 8.75% higher and their high-density lipoproteins correspondingly 16.6% higher, their low-density lipoproteins (usually considered the undesirable ones) were only 0.60% higher. (The very low-density ones were still higher.) Body weights only increased 2.7% and they appeared in good health.

Today, eating high quantities of fat is looked upon by some people as unhealthy. On the other hand, certain unsaturated fats, such as the three-omega unsaturated fatty acids that are found in fish living in cooler waters, are considered beneficial for preventing arteriosclerosis.[16] Stefansson, a man of many facets, was the one person who tried to bring the foods and habits of the people of the north to the armchairs and living rooms of most of us. Stefansson's main claim, however, was not that pemmican was an excellent food, but that active individuals could maintain good health on a raw or slightly cooked all-meat or all-fish diet.

Stefansson may be remembered with mixed feelings. He did not have a powerful backer or adversary to arouse the press, like Peary with the backing of the Explorers Club and the United States Navy, or Cook with the scorn of Peary. If he had, perhaps there would be more interest in him. As it is, he is more apt to be forgotten, fading into an arctic mist.

Notes

1. Nancy Fogelson, *Arctic Exploration & International Relations 1900–1932* (Fairbanks: University of Alaska Press, 1992), 61.

2. V. Stefansson, *The Friendly Arctic* (New York: Macmillan Co., 1921); *Hunters of the Great North* (New York: Harcourt, Brace and Co., 1944); and *Not by Bread Alone* (New York: Macmillan Co., 1946).

3. V. Stefansson, *Hunters of the Great North*, 1.

4. Fogelson, *Arctic Exploration & International Relations*, 65.

5. B. Lopez, *Arctic Dreams, Imagination and Desire in a Northern Landscape* (New York: Charles Scribner's Sons, 1986), 387.

6. See Lopez, *Arctic Dreams*, and Stefansson, *The Friendly Arctic*, 7.

7. Stefansson, *Hunters of the Great North*, 69.

8. Stefansson, *The Friendly Arctic*, 480.

9. Stefansson, *Not by Bread Alone*, 60.

10. In reading the pros and cons in these fights today, and they were fights, the points raised from both sides not only seem peculiar but sometimes just wrong. But back then, those on each side considered their information, ideas and arguments completely valid. Stefansson thought ice-cold water was thrown on his beliefs without paying any attention to what people actually ate in the icy north.

11. For example, I started my Ph.D. training in biochemistry at the University of Wisconsin in 1938, then a Mecca of vitamin discoveries. There, Stefansson was not only ridiculed, but his arguments and research were not considered worthy of attention. I left there highly prejudiced.

12. For one year of the third expedition, Karsten Andersen, a young Dane, had eaten just meat and water. It is also important to note that for several years he worked on his own Florida orange grove; he lived outside, away from the cold, and his diet was high in vegetables and fruit.

13. Stefansson, *Not by Bread Alone*, 275.

14. R. M. Kark, R. E. Johnson, and J. S. Lewis, "Defects of Pemmican as an Emergency Ration for Infantry Troops," *War Medicine* 7 (1945): 345–352.

15. W. Steger and P. Schurke, *North to the Pole* (New York: Ivy Books, 1987), 294.

16. W. G. Linscher and A. J. Bergroesen, "Lipids," in *Modern Nutrition in Health and Disease*, M. E. Shils and V. R. Young, eds. (Philadelphia: Lea and Feiger, 1988), 289.

12

In To the South Pacific
and On To Antarctica

The South Pacific for some has carried with it ideas and fantasies of wealth, romance, and the attraction of searching for the unknown. During the 18th century and well in to the 19th, early explorers pursued these ideas. Magellan's voyage and the subsequent dozen voyages by others up to the middle 1750s did a lot to dispel ignorance about the area and to provide knowledge about the people who lived there. Few were interested in Antarctica.

The earlier period of horrible nutritional problems aboard southern-going ships might be considered to have nearly ended with the explorations of George Anson who, from 1740–1744, had five ships going to the South Pacific.[1] In crossing the Atlantic, flies, fleas, and rats were his company, and eventually dysentery and scurvy. After rounding Cape Horn he returned to England; of the 1,900 men who had set sail with him, he lost 1,145. Greater than ninety percent of these deaths were caused by disease, and over half, 997, were from scurvy. In contrast was Commodore Byron's expedition from 1764 to 1766 in the South Pacific. He enforced hygiene and also had live animals aboard for food, as well as generous quantities of onions in the diet. None of his crew experienced symptoms of scurvy.

French expeditions also were usually under their navy. As was their custom, wine and other alcoholic drinks were major provisions.[2] In reports, the French Navy's rations in the 18th century were ample, supplying about 4,000 calories. In practice, however, they were at best only fair, and usually poor. They provided two pounds of solid rations along with nearly a liter of wine or other drinks containing an equivalent amount of alcohol. Also, although ships were not usually underprovisioned, starvation nevertheless occurred because the food was poorly selected and became inedible from extensive deterioration. Microbial growth, insect infestation, and chemical changes undoubtedly all occurred extensively. As always, these problems

Table 12.1

Recorded overall losses in Anson's squadron—a conservative estimate[a,b]

Deaths from fevers and dysentery	320
Deaths from scurvy	997
Deaths from starvation and exposure	35
Abandoned - presumed deaths from starvation	19
Deaths from accident (plus accidents at Cape Horn)	9+
Deaths from action (Payta and Covadonga)	4
Murdered	4
Deserted	10
Other (including deaths from China or Rio to England)	17
Total	**1415**

a. George Anson's circumnavigation was from 1741 to 1744.

b. From J. Watt, E. J. Freeman, and W. F. Bynum, eds., *Starving Sailors: The Influence of Nutrition upon Naval and Maritime History* (London: National Maritime Museum, 1981).

were made worse by the inadequacy of proper provisioning due to administrative errors and the dishonesty of suppliers and officers.

Two of the more famous expeditions were by the French leader Louis Antoine de Bougainville, a captain in the French Navy, and by Captain James Cook of the British Navy. Bougainville was one of the most educated of ship captains of his time, and probably one of the most humane.[3] A former lawyer, a mathematician, an army officer with service in Canada, and an author of two published books, he wrote that there was usually no consideration for the health of soldiers or seamen. Then he had to contend with the French bureaucracy. Although he was a fine leader, Bougainville's expedition was in general an unsuccessful one. His voyage from 1766 to 1769 was probably a good example of how poor planning by administrators can result in near disaster. In addition to the projected explorations, the ship had French government administrative stops to make, which greatly lengthened the time of their voyages. And then they had a poor choice of a ship, the *Boudeuse*. Although it was a new ship of 900 tons, it had over 200 passengers and crew aboard and could not carry nearly enough food to supply these people for very long. As a result, they had to have a supply ship. Many things went wrong, including extensive rotting of the foods in the tropical areas, difficulties in meeting with the supply ship, and when the supply ship was met, food on that was also rotten. Fortunately there were many rats eating the rotting food, and by eating rats a good supply of vitamin C could be obtained, at least for those able to purchase them from the rat catchers. Indeed, even the poultry they had taken aboard suffered because one of the main foods they were given was bananas, and poultry died on such a diet. Bananas did not help the crew either, because they are only a fair source of vitamin C.

It was on November 15, 1766, that Bougainville left Nantes, but it wasn't until November 14 a year later that he weighed anchor at Montevideo and not until April 4, 1768, that he arrived at Tahiti. Arriving at Buru on September 1, Bougainville stated that in a little over a week's further sailing there would have been many deaths, and poor health in most of the rest of the crew. There was plenty of food, but it was either rotten food or the wrong kind of food. The rotten food, however, may have indirectly helped decrease the severity of scurvy, because the rats ate the food and the men ate the rats, synthesizers of lots of vitamin C.

To sea-borne explorers and those interested in the nutrition and health of seamen, the three voyages of Captain James Cook stand forth as the most productive and successful of the 1700s. From 1768 to 1779 he headed three great voyages in the South Pacific, even to the ice-ridden waters in Antarctica and to the northern areas off Alaska, seeking the polar passage.[4]

He proved conclusively that long ocean voyages were not incompatible with good health. Although there were deaths from infectious diseases and even from cannibalistic natives on the islands, he did not lose a man from malnutrition. After some problems with his first voyage, his record thereafter was nearly perfect. He chose ships that were capable of going into shallow waters, thereby allowing exploration of coastlines and the capability of landing to procure fresh foods. He sought fresh foods with great vigor, particularly edible greenstuffs such as wild celery, scurvy grass, winter's bark, cresses, berries, and spruce needles. Beaglehole describes Cook's intense activity on landing at the southern coast of New Zealand:

> Tents were pitched near the stream for the water, coopers, sailmakers, the forge was set up for the repair of iron work; the fishermen were out every day; Cook began to brew "spruce beer" on the Newfoundland model when the leaves and small branches of a tree which he thought 'resembles the American Black Spruce'—the New Zealand rimu—together with those of the less astringent 'tea shrub' or manuka, his inspissated Juice of Wort and molasses. The majority of the crew took to it very well. Indeed, they had to, for when the beer was started the spirits were stopped. Cook thought it was healthful and a fair substitute for the green vegetables of which he could here find none.[5]

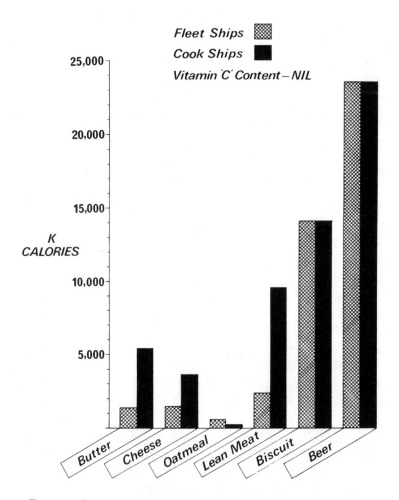

Energy yield per man per week. Alcohol made the largest contribution to energy requirements of the 18th century sailor. J. Watt, 1981

Yet on Cook's first trip, when he was learning, forty-one of the ship's complement of ninety-four died, and thirty-one of these deaths were from malaria and dysentery. Although three men developed scurvy, no one died from it. One wonders, however, whether some of the cases of dysentery had been aggravated by scurvy.

After these experiences Cook embarked on his great 60,000 mile voyage, which lasted from 1772 to 1775. He went with two ships, the *Resolution*, which he captained, and the *Adventure*. Only four crew died on the *Resolution*, one from tuberculosis and three from other causes. However, on the *Adventure* three died. On both ships Cook demanded that the crew practice stringent health rules.

Life aboard the *Adventure* was not as healthful as on the *Resolution*. At one time:

> Then the *Adventure's* men began to go down with scurvy. Our cook, a dirty hinterland man, a natural prey, died of it on 23 July, though Cook learned nothing of sickness for five days more. He was able to send a boat on board the day after that and was told that 26 men were sick with scurvy and flux. He immediately dispatched a new cook and used every method he could think of on Furneaux, the captain, to stay the disease. A few of his own crew were showing slight symptoms, but they were already being specially dieted...However, in spite of Cook's demand for frequent provisioning of the ships with fresh plant material and any other animal or birds that could be found, he was a subscriber to the advocacy of wort and malt. Although his diet appeared nutritionally better than that of the general fleet ships, particularly insofar as containing butter and cheese and lean meat, it was generally devoid of vitamin C and generously endowed with beer.[6]

Of the total calories per man per day, over forty percent came from beer.[7] Of course, beer was a morale sustainer as well as a food, and morale sustainers were necessary, perhaps even aiding appetites for a less desirable diet. At best, however, only frequent inhabitants of bars or pubs would term it a healthful dietary constituent. Hamstrung by naval traditions and the customs and beliefs of the times, Cook nevertheless appears to us today as a good practical nutritionist.

Alcohol was common at Cook's time and keeps cropping up again and again in most other early descriptions. As might be expected, the customs of the times were also followed by U.S. ships. On Cook's third voyage searching for the passage across the arctic region from Alaska east, his record was not as good as the first one, and unfortunately he was killed by natives in the Hawaiian Islands.[8]

Nevertheless, he had forged ahead along a pathway that many future explorers ought to have followed, but unfortunately frequently did not. Cook's successes were probably due in great measure to his strong appreciation of fresh foods, this apparently without knowing the value of Dr. Lind's much earlier discoveries. Yet, he proclaimed the importance of malt and wort, essentially useless for treating or preventing scurvy. Perhaps his very successes also retarded the adoption of Lind's recommendations. But here was a person who, with good planning, a reasonably open mind, common sense, and the demand for discipline, showed how nutritional deficiencies could be largely prevented.

By the middle of the 19th century, and very much so by its end, nutritional problems on ships had become much easier to handle. One principal reason was that the use of steam shortened the times at sea. Another was an increase in the number of ports-of-call with facilities for resupply and, of course, a better knowledge of the causes of food spoilage. An English surgeon, Sir Alexander Armstrong, in 1858 summarized his beliefs on scurvy aboard ships:

> Towards the close of the last century the channel fleet was unable to keep at sea and the squadron under the command of Lord Geary in 1780 returned to England with twenty-four hundred men afflicted with scurvy.
> The disease continued to prevail in the fleet for several years subsequently to a greater or lesser extent and it was not until fifteen years after the return

Table 12.2
Basic ship's provisions of the British Royal Navy before 1800[a,b]

Day	Biscuit	Beer	Beef	Pork	Peas	Oatmeal	Butter[c]	Cheese[c]
	(lb)	(gal)	(lb)	(lb)	(pt)	(pt)	(oz)	(oz)
Sunday	1	1	-	1	1/2	-	2	-
Monday	1	1	-	-	-	1	2	4
Tuesday	1	1	2	-	-	-	-	-
Wednesday	1	1	-	-	1/2	1	2	4
Thursday	1	1	-	1	1/2	-	-	-
Friday	1	1	-	-	1/2	1	2	4
Saturday	1	1	2	-	-	-	-	-

[a]Added later (in 1808) were 6 oz. of sugar a week and fresh vegetables when available in a port and when money was available.
[b]From Lloyd and Coulter (1961a).
[c]Unfortunately, at times butter and cheese might be omitted.

of Admiral Geary, namely in 1795, that any means was adapted for improving the health and presenting the occurrence of this terrible scourge— Although the remedy (lime juice) had long been known, yet it was not until this period that it was officially ordered to be supplied to the Navy.

Since the disease had therefore almost disappeared from the Navy, it is only to the polar voyages that we must look for the reoccurrence of scurvy— All expeditions had scurvy and deaths, except for one in the unprecedentedly long period, to which I have alluded, occurred aboard the HMS Investigator during the latter's expedition to the polar regions. In the following pages I shall attempt to account for the immunity from this disease, which was enjoyed by no other ship.

The lemon juice with which we were supplied was of the most excellent quality and was of two kinds, one which was prepared by adding a tenth part of brandy and the other was simply boiled, containing no spirits. The juice was kept in bottles containing 64 oz. with a level of olive oil about one half inch on the surface and the bottles were carefully corked and sealed. In pursuance of this plan, it was carefully mixed in separate tubs from which each man daily drank his allowance in the presence of an officer. To this circumstance, I am therefore not hesitant to attribute not only the immunity we enjoyed from scurvy for a longer time than had ever been known in the polar sea—But although lemon juice is regularly issued it does not follow that it is consumed.[9]

The end of the 19th century brought one of the first major probes into Antarctica and the first wintering-over there. It did not come from the major powers or the Scandinavian experts; it came from Belgium. A naval officer, Lt. Adrien de Gerlache, mounted his own expedition, obtained money from many sources, bought a ship named the *Belgica*, and got hold of the two veteran arctic explorers, Roald Amundsen and Frederick Cook.[10] Leaving Antwerp the end of August 1897, the *Belgica*, with a complement of nineteen, sailed initially for the east coast of South America and then into the area surrounding the Antarctic Peninsula. Lt. de Gerlache's intent was then to circle around to Cape Adare (due south of New Zealand), and to be the first explorer to winter over in Antarctica. The ambition was there, but his planning was not equal to the ambition. The ship was provisioned with inadequate clothing and a mixture of many types of food which de Gerlache's crew, from different lands and cultures, had trouble eating. The ship became frozen in the ice and drifted for many months; it was not until March of 1899 that the *Belgica* was seen again, sailing into Punta Arenas, Chile.

Cook probably saved the expedition from a serious problem with scurvy. His preventative remedy for scurvy resulted from his arctic experience and his believing that fresh meat was the answer. This led to his recommendation to supply the men with penguin meat. De Gerlache disagreed with the choice of food but, nevertheless, finally allowed a large number of penguins to be killed and frozen.

By the end of May, near the height of the antarctic winter, the need for fresh meat became alarming to Cook, who wrote:

> We ate little, however, and were thoroughly disgusted with canned foods. We had tried the meat of the penguins, but to the majority its flavour was still too [fishy]. We entered the long night somewhat underfed, not because there was a scarcity of food, but because of our unconquerable dislike for such as we had. It is possible to support life for seven or eight months upon a diet of canned food; but after this period there is something in the human system which makes it refuse to utilize the elements of nutrition contained in tins. Against such food, even for a short period, the stomach protests; confined to it for a long period, it simply refuses to exercise its functions. Articles which in the canning retain a natural appearance usually remain, especially if cooked a little, friendly to the palate. This is particularly true of meat retaining hard fibers, such as ham, bacon, dried meats, and corned beef. It is also true of fruits preserved in juices; and vegetables, such as peas, corn, tomatoes, and of dried things. Unfortunately this class of food formed a small part of our store. We were weighed down with the supposed finer delicacies of the Belgian, French, and Norwegian markets. We had laboratory mixtures in neat cans, combined in such a manner as to make them look tempting—hashes under various catchy names; sausage stuffs in deceptive forms, meat and fishballs said to contain cream, mysterious soups, and all the latest inventions in condensed foods. But they one and all proved failures, as a steady diet. The stomach demands things with a natural fiber, or some tough, gritty substance. At this time, as a relief, we would have taken kindly to something containing pebbles or sand. How we longed to use our teeth![11]

And a little later he wrote:

> We are all eating appreciably less now than during the bright season—and either there is a constant inclination to sleep or persistent insomnia. We eat an amount of fat, however, that would surprise most people; fat pork, fatty meats, the pure oil of bacon, and tremendous quantities of oleomargarine, are consumed with apparent relish. This is to me particularly surprising because during three arctic voyages I never noticed any particular craving for fat; but this I ascribe to the fact that we always ate liberally of fresh meats north, and these we have not here. We eat a little penguin with a show of pleasure, but most of us are quite tired of its marine flavour and fish-oil smoothness. If we had sufficient ham it would afford immense gastric delight. There is much indigestion now—fermentation, gastric inertia, intestinal and gastric pain, imperfect hepatic action, and a general suppression of all the digestive secretions.[12]

Cook went further in recommending penguin steaks to most who became ill, particularly when what Cook called "polar anemia" appeared. In

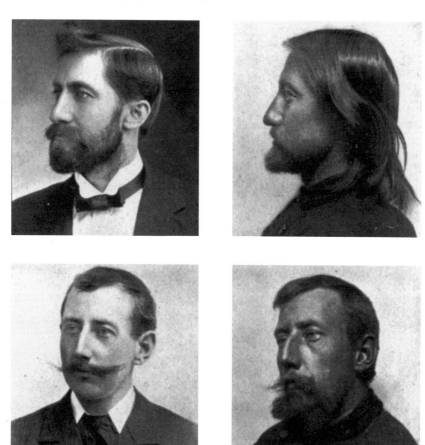

How Frederick Cook (top) and Roald Amundsen (bottom) looked before and after the
Belgica expedition. "We were all reasonably good-looking when we embarked, but we
were otherwise when we returned. The long night effected a radical transformation
in our physiognomies." F. A. Cook, 1900

one case, when he was treating the captain of the ship, Georges Lecointe,
he described the treatment and situation in this way:

> The first upon whom I tried this system of treatment systematically was
> Lecointe. I had urged part of it upon Daco, but he could not eat the pen-
> guin, and when I told him he must, he said he would rather die. When
> Lecointe came under treatment I told him that if he would follow the
> treatment carefully I thought he would be out of bed in a week. I did not
> have this faith in the treatment at that time, but I had confidence in the

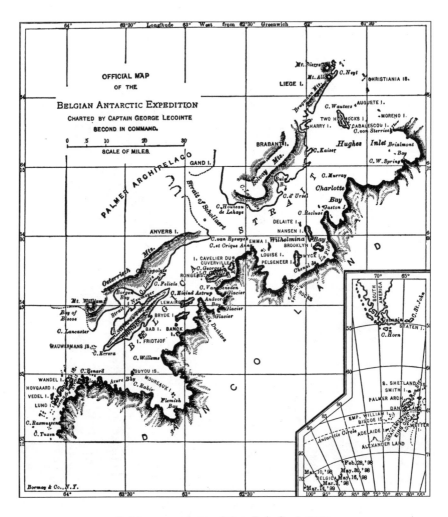

Belgian antarctic expedition. F. A. Cook, 1900

soundness of Lecointe's organs and I wished to boon up the man. Lecointe replied by saying, 'I will sit on the stove for a month and eat penguins for the rest of my polar life if that will do me good.'[13]

In his diary dated July 17, 1898, Cook summarized the value of his fresh penguin meat by writing, "If we had not fresh (frozen) meat to eat and an abundance of fuel to give heat, I'm sure we would have an alarming mortality in less than a month. Several lives have certainly been saved eating penguins, and we shall always owe them a debt of gratitude."[14] In the *Belgica* there was still a supply of canned meats when they left Antarctica.

Perhaps Dr. Cook overemphasized the value of fresh penguin meat because there must have been some vitamin C in some of the canned foods, but still he kept the crew from crossing the line leading to a condition of scurvy and other nutritional or digestive problems. But some of the explorers yet to travel to Antarctica did not rely heavily on Cook's ideas. Could this be because they did not believe his reports on his northern explorations? But Amundsen seemed to trust Cook's medical ideas, perhaps helping Amundsen maintain good nutrition on his two future successful polar trips.

Adventure, money, fame, and national pride brought many others to Antarctica during the end of the 19th century and into the first decade of the 20th. Either directly or indirectly most interlocked with the succeeding expeditions of Scott and Amundsen.

Representing the enterprising Norwegians, C. A. Larsen in 1892 and 1893 was on the islands off the Antarctic Peninsula and on the east coast itself. An excellent whaler but not an explorer, he did very well. In a true Robert Scott tradition, he brought home samples of fossil wood and fossil bivalves, outstanding discoveries for the time. In 1901, the Swedish sent O. H. Nordenskjold to dig further into C. A. Larsen's discoveries of the fossils. Not only did Nordenskjold do this but he added the evidence that the antarctic mountain range of the peninsula was an extension of the Andes. Wintering over and a shipwreck caused separations and difficulties, but penguins and seals probably saved them from scurvy (perhaps they were fortunate in being far enough north and with good weather to facilitate the capture of these as food). Dr. Jean Charcot, son of the famous French neurophysiologist Dr. Jean Martin Charcot, sailed under the French flag in 1903 and again in 1908 along the Antarctic Peninsula. Perhaps he is mainly remembered for a publicized friendly relationship with Scott, a welcome bond between France and England. In 1911, Germany was there through the expedition of Wilhem Filchner. Heading for the Weddell Sea, on the side of Antarctica opposite to Scott's planned-for target of the Ross Sea for his trip in 1911, he had Scott's approval. Drifting and tossing for the winter, the expedition could not land, but reportedly did not suffer malnutrition. Sea life should have been available.

Not many nonscientists remember the exploits of Carstens Borchgrevink, a Norwegian sailing under an English flag.[15] His quiet and relatively uneventful expedition in 1898, however, had a first: a well planned over-wintering in a prefabricated house on Cape Adare, farther south than ever before. The scientists made highly important physical and biological

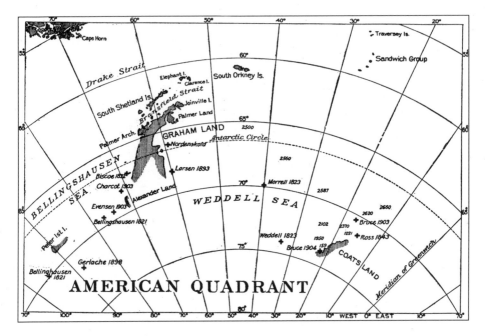

The American quadrant of the antarctic expedition before 1910. A. W. Greely, 1910

observations.[16] All went well nutritionally with an orderly menu supplemented with seal and penguin meat. Borchgrevink wrote: "Seal beef and roasted penguin flesh became later a frequent repast, as we grew frightfully tired of tinned food."[17] The menu was a good one for the knowledge accepted then, but would have been inadequate alone. Lucky for them that they tired of the canned food, for the seal and penguin meat probably steered them away from some scurvy.

Borchgrevink's menus were well planned to provide some variations, but on a repetitive weekly basis. Breakfast always had porridge (cereal) and bread and butter with ham, bacon, or cheese. Lunches had cheese plus tongue, herrings plus sardines and cheese, or ham and cheese. Dinners were perhaps not as varied with potatoes of some type and usually tinned fish or salted meat. Vegetables (dry) were only served twice a week at dinner, but a milk soup (recipe not given) was served three times. Cocoa was an everyday item. Forays for supplemental foods heightened the nutritional values and made the menus more acceptable.

Combining well-planned diets and menus with forays from the house as headquarters, Borchgrevink supplied his men with physical activity and sufficient nutrition.

Notes

1. J. Watt, "Some consequences of nutritional disorders in 18th century British circumnavigations," in *Starving Sailors: The Influence of Nutrition upon Naval and Maritime History*, J. Watt, E. J. Freeman, and W. F. Bynum, eds. (London: National Maritime Museum, 1981), 51.
2. A. Carre, "Eighteenth-century French voyages of exploration: general problems of nutrition with special reference to the voyages of Bougainville and d'Entrecasteaux," in *Starving Sailors: The Influence of Nutrition upon Naval and Maritime History*, 73–84.
3. Ibid.
4. J. C. Beaglehole, *The Life of Captain James Cook* (Stanford: Stanford University Press, 1974); B. Hooper, ed., *With Captain Cook in the Antarctic and Pacific. The Private Journal of James Burney* (Canberra: National Library of Australia, 1975).
5. Beaglehole, *The Life of Captain James Cook*, 324.
6. Ibid., 338.
7. J. Watt, "Some consequences of nutritional disorders in eighteenth-century British circumnavigations," 51.
8. Ibid., 676. When a bundle of Cook's remains were given to the ship's crew, it contained the scalp, all the long bones, thighs, legs, arms, and the skull, all of which were scraped clean.
9. He goes on to say that even in navy ships the lemon juice may not be consumed, but this is even more so on merchant ships. In addition, the lemon juices on merchant ships may be of poor quality and diluted with ineffective acids. A. Armstrong, *Observations on Naval Hygiene and Scurvy, More Particularily as the Latter Appeared During a Polar Voyage* (London: J. Churchill, 1858).
10. F. A. Cook, *Through the First Antarctic Night* (New York: Doubleday and McClure Co., 1900), x.
11. Ibid., 302.
12. Ibid., 306.
13. Ibid., 333. He did sit beside the stove two hours daily for a month, and he ate, by his own choosing, penguin steaks for the balance of his stay in the polar circle. In a week he was about, and in a fortnight he again made his observations, and for the rest of his polar existence he was again one of the strongest men on the *Belgica*.
14. Ibid., 334.
15. C. E. Borchgrevink, *First on the Arctic Continent* (Montreal: McGill-Queen's University Press, 1962), 1.
16. The author has spent over a quarter of a century studying the proteins of an antarctic fish named for Carstens Borchgrevink (Feeney, 1974). This fish is *Trematomas borchgrevinki*.
17. Borchgrevink, *First on the Arctic Continent*, 153.

13

First Expeditions in Antarctica: Amundsen, Mawson, Shackleton, and Scott

Robert Falcon Scott, Roald Amundsen, Douglas Mawson, and Ernest Shackleton—major figures in the conquest of Antarctica—had their differences,[1] but they also had many characteristics in common: they were resolute, serious, conscientious, hard-working men, able to endure fatigue and pain. All four planned their expeditions in detail, though each ended with different degrees of success and suffering. All four were very concerned about the food and nutrition for themselves and their men.

Douglas Mawson was a member of Shackleton's second polar attempt, who then in 1912 conducted a survey of western Antarctica where he lost two of his men and nearly died, apparently from hypervitaminosis A, after eating dog liver. Ernest Shackleton first went to Antarctica in 1901 with Scott in an unsuccessful attempt to reach the South Pole. Shackleton tried again unsuccessfully in 1908 as leader of his own group, and in 1914–1916, he planned to make a 1,600-mile transantarctic march via the pole, but instead he was forced to make some of the greatest sea voyages in small boats. Robert Falcon Scott and Roald Amundsen competed at nearly the same time in 1911 for the race to the South Pole, with different procedures and outcomes; Scott arrived a month after Amundsen and then died with his four companions on the return trip, while Amundsen returned with his team well and hearty.

Of the four explorers, Shackleton was the most colorful; he made the most trips, traveled the farthest in Antarctica, and led his men to safety on the longest ride in small boats in antarctic history without starvation or loss of life. An Anglo-Irishman who loved poetry, Shackleton went to sea at age sixteen in the merchant marine. At twenty-seven he joined Scott's first antarctic expedition, a tough, active man, but with a carefully hidden heart

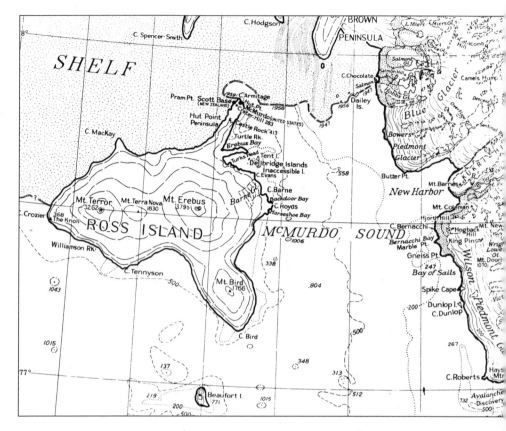

Map of Ross Island. National Science Foundation

murmur. This murmur probably was the forerunner of his death by a heart attack nearly twenty years later.

Scott was a traditional British Navy career officer who believed rules were to be followed absolutely.[2] On Christmas Eve of 1901 Scott left Lyttelton, New Zealand, on the official National Antarctic Expedition to probe toward the South Pole—his first polar exploration. Long before this departure, much preparation and planning had been done, not all of which proved to be the most prudent for a successful expedition. On the positive side, Scott obtained considerable advice and assistance from northern polar explorers and from many other craftsmen and seamen. His ship, the *Discovery*, designed by an admiralty shipwright, was specially constructed for traveling through the ice.[3] Although reinforced to withstand the ice, fully loaded it did not handle the polar voyage well.[4]

With the voyage to Antarctica accomplished, Scott set up his base on Ross Island at McMurdo Sound near the Ross Ice Shelf, a place they named Hut Point. Here he and his crew spent the late spring and winter preparing for the onslaught to the pole the following antarctic spring. They had extensive equipment but, according to many observers and writers, little knowledge of its use. Most did not know how to ski, and the dogs had no trainer; even more important, the dogs never became accustomed to the leaders. It was a seemingly small matter to Scott, yet any good dog handler knew the importance of a well-developed relationship between dogs and their owners.

Some of the early trips prior to the dash for the south should have given Scott forebodings of future serious problems with scurvy. After one trip on which Lieutenant A. B. Armitage and Surgeon Reginald Kettlitz reported, Scott was shocked on hearing that they had suffered from scurvy:

> The result of Wilson's medical examination of this party on their return has been handed to me; the gist of it is that Heald, Mr. Ferrar and Cross have very badly swollen legs, whilst Heald's are discoloured as well. Heald and Cross have also swollen and spongy gums. The remainder of the party seem fairly well, but not above suspicion; Walker's ankles are slightly swollen.... Though there is not much else but scurvy in my thoughts just at present, the great thing is to pretend that there is nothing to be alarmed at....[5]

Scott took various precautions to prevent scurvy. He ordered a general housecleaning, possibly due to his naval training as well as to some current beliefs that sanitation and wholesome living conditions prevented scurvy. Added to this was the belief that canned meats could contain a poisonous agent, rooted in the ptomaine theory that spoilage caused scurvy. He also believed that lemon juice would not prevent scurvy.[6] Thus, Scott's preparations and plannings for the polar trip (as well as his disastrous trip nearly a decade later) were not based on the best nutritional concepts, and he relied on rations only slightly upgraded from those of far earlier expeditions. He summarized these unfortunate beliefs:

> For centuries, and until quite recently, it was believed that the antidote to scurvy lay in vegetable acids; scurvy grass was sought by the older voyages, and finally lime-juice was made, and remains, a legal necessity for ships travelling on the high seas. Behind this belief lies a vast amount of evidence, but a full consideration of this evidence is beset with immense difficulties. For instance, although it is an undoubted fact that with the introduction of lime-juice scurvy was largely diminished, yet is apt to be forgotten that there were other causes which might have contributed to this

result; for at the same time sea voyages were being largely reduced by steam power, and owners were forced to provide much better food for their men....

I understand that scurvy is now believed to be ptomaine poisoning, caused by the virus of the bacterium of decay in meat, and in plain language, as long as a man continues to assimilate this poison he is bound to get worse, and when he ceases to add to the quantity taken the system tends to throw it off, and the patient recovers. The practical point, therefore, is to obtain meat which does not contain this poison, and herein lies the whole difficulty of the case, for danger lurks everywhere. Tainted fresh meat may be virulent, but in the ordinary course of events one eats it rarely and so is saved from any disastrous result. The risk of a taint in tinned meat is greater because of the process involved in its manufacture, and with salt meat the risk is greater still for the same reason. To what extent meat must be tainted to produce scurvy is unknown, but there is reason to suppose that the taint can be so slight as to escape the notice of one's senses; in other words, poison may lurk in a tin of meat which to the sight, taste, and smell appears to be in perfect condition. Such a supposition alone shows the difficulty of tracing an outbreak of the disease to its exact source....

It has been pointed out that scurvy depends largely on environment, and there can be no doubt that severe or insanitary conditions of life contribute to the ravages of the disease. Indeed, we saw how this might be from the outbreak in our western party, but I do not think such conditions can be regarded as the prime cause.[7]

According to Scott's listings, his daily rations for the polar trip contained 8.6 ounces of protein, 4.4 ounces of fat and 15.6 ounces of carbohydrate. This calculates to be about 3,500 calories. The amount of food (in ounces) carried per day, per man, as originally outlined by Scott was: biscuit, 12.0; oatmeal, 1.5; pemmican, 7.6; rad ration, 1.1; plasmon (meat concentrate), 2.0; pea flour, 1.5; cheese, 2.0; chocolate, 1.1; cocoa, 0.7; sugar, 3.8. In addition, small quantities of tea, onion powder, pepper and salt were available. In spite of Scott's eventual serious food problems, he deserves much credit for his attention to the rations and actual eating on his expedition.[8]

He carefully compared his daily allowance of 35.5 ounces with those of Greely (36 oz.), McClintock (42 oz.), Nares (40 oz.), and Parry in his early days (20 oz.), noting that Parry's sledging trips were short and that his party still must have been famished.

On November 2, 1902, Scott, Wilson, and Shackleton set off for the pole with a team of nineteen dogs.[9] Problems soon ensued, particularly for the dogs. Shackleton, unaware that a dog's natural gait is a trot, pushed them too hard. Compounding the problem, he did not plan well for their food. Apparently they were fed only dog biscuits most of the winter. Some critics

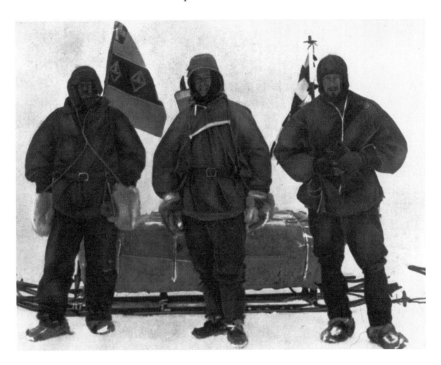

The southern party of Scott, left to right: E. H. Shackleton, R. F. Scott, E. A. Wilson.
R. F. Scott, 1905

have stated that these dog biscuits were supposed to be supplemented with meat and not offered alone.

Before long the dogs were pulling poorly, and by the end of the southern probe, not a single dog was alive. The dogs were not killed just to provide meat for the living ones. They either died or they were killed when they became incapacitated. This unfortunate and unnecessary experience with dogs greatly colored the future expeditions of both Shackleton and Scott and may have been responsible for the death of Scott and his four companions on his later expedition.

Soon the men were on restricted rations and antagonisms developed between Scott and Shackleton. Edmund Wilson tried to maintain peace between them with some success, but it was not sufficient to quench the jealousy, rivalry, and perhaps even a little hatred. On reaching 82.17° south on December 31, they turned back. The return trip was a horrible one; reaching each base camp was a struggle as they became desperate for food. Scott's diary is replete with their dreams and their thoughts as they marched along, and most every one was of food. In one entry, for example, the men stopped at a food depot only to discover it was not well stocked. They searched every nook and cranny for any possible items, however small, that might have been dropped on the trek towards the pole. Of those they found, Scott's share was a small piece of biscuit. He relished this tiny relic of the outward trip like a tray of party food.

Their problems were compounded by scurvy. Scurvy had actually developed among the whole crew at Hut Point over two months before they started. Perhaps the crew was already suffering from borderline nutritional deficiencies even before embarking on the journey as the British diet for working people was poor at that time; nutritional inadequacies followed many men going to sea. All three suffered from it, but Shackleton the worst. He eventually became incapacitated for a period and he rode on the sled that the other two men pulled. Scott wrote:

> January 14. This morning we had a thorough medical examination, and the result was distinctly unsatisfactory. Shackleton has very angry-looking gums—swollen and dark; he is also suffering greatly from shortness of breath; his throat seems to be congested, and he gets fits of coughing, when he is obliged to spit, and once or twice to-day he has spat blood. I myself have distinctly red gums, and a very slight swelling in the ankles. Wilson's gums are affected in one spot, where there is a large plum-coloured lump; other-wise he seems free from symptoms. Both he and I feel quite fit and well, and as far as we are concerned I think a breakdown is very far removed.[10]

Nevertheless, Shackleton struggled on, and soon resumed all activities, even doing more than his share by the end. By this time, however, the tension between Scott and Shackleton was obvious. When they were almost back to Hut Point, Scott recognized their general poor state:

> That it is none too soon is evident. We are as near spent as three persons can well be. If Shackleton has shown a temporary improvement, we know by experience how little confidence we can place in it, and how near he has been and still is to a total collapse. As for Wilson and myself, we have scarcely liked to known how 'done' we are, and how greatly the last week or two has tried us. We have known that our scurvy has been advancing again with rapid strides, but as we could do nothing more to prevent it, we have not looked beyond the signs that have made themselves obvious. Wilson has suffered from lameness for many a day; the cause was plain, and we knew it must increase. Each morning he has vainly attempted to disguise a limp, and his set face has shown me that there is much to be gone through before the first stiffness wears off. As for myself, for some time I have hur-ried through the task of changing my foot-gear in an attempt to forget that

my ankles are considerably swollen. One and all we want rest and peace, and, all being well, to-morrow, thank Heaven, we shall get them.[11]

On returning to Hut Point on February 3, Scott declared that Shackleton would have to be evacuated for illness. Many have wondered whether this was his true assessment, or whether it was due to their mutual antagonism. This rebuff was taken as a mortal blow by Shackleton, and he never forgave Scott. The great fatigue plus the evident symptoms of scurvy leave no doubt that all three men suffered from a vitamin C deficiency, and possibly other deficiencies. Making it back alive, they had struggled again and again because of lack of food. They had been gone ninety-three days; Shackleton had clinical scurvy after seventy-three. Assuming that their bodily stores of vitamin C were low before they started and the vitamin C content of their trail rations was also low, one might expect their outbreak of scurvy.

Whether Scott's decision to send Ernest Shackleton home as an invalid increased Shackleton's ambition for returning to Antarctica and making an attempt at the pole is only speculation. Still, only two or three years after returning from the polar exploit with Scott, Shackleton made the attempt, organizing his own expedition.[12] Everyone knew he was competing with Scott, especially Scott himself. Obtaining financing was very difficult for Shackleton. Everyone was critical, thinking he might be using Scott's former travel route, Scott foremost among those with such thoughts. Scott was on a battleship far from England when he learned about Shackleton's proposed trip. Perhaps it was the battleship atmosphere that caused him to write a note to Shackleton to the effect that only through ignorance could he expect Shackleton to be attempting to go to Antarctica, knowing that Scott already had plans to return. In his answer, Shackleton ended by saying, "Especially I think my desires were as great, if not greater, than anyone else's to return, seeing that I was cut off by a premature return to this country from further participation in the expedition."[13] After several exchanges Shackleton finally wrote Scott that he would not go to McMurdo Sound but would find a route elsewhere. Thus, old wounds, memories, and ambitions set the course for another mad dash to the South Pole.

On New Year's Day of 1908 Shackleton's ship, the *Nimrod*, left New Zealand with a tremendous send-off by the New Zealanders. His shore party consisted of eleven men, with the later addition of L. A. Mackintosh. Of the twelve men, three had journeyed with Shackleton before. Two of them—Lt. J. B. Adams, RNR, and Frank Wild—accompanied him, along with Dr. Eric Marshall, on his final polar dash. Unfortunately a cloud descended upon them that was never wholly lifted throughout Shackleton's life. Probing other possible landings and locations for his main base and finding these undesirable, he finally settled on Ross Island, McMurdo Sound, the place Scott, and much of the world, believed belonged to Scott. A deadly sin had been committed. The base camp was set up at Cape Royds, about thirty miles north of Scott's previous hut of the *Discovery* expedition. Here they wintered over, making ready for the antarctic spring take-off. They had dogs, but they did not use them. They also had eight ponies, but only four survived and made the start to the pole. Again poor luck, or perhaps poor judgment, interfered, as the ponies had been quartered on a salty, sandy area, and three of them had died from eating the sand from want of salt, while a fourth died from poisoning due to exposure to waste. Ponies also needed extra roughage and were gravely effected by the cold, by sweating, by freezing of the accumulated sweat, and by being unable to curl up like dogs in a fur ball in the snow.

Certainly they could have done better without their cantankerous motor sledge. Although it was functional for laying down the initial depot, the sledge only bored itself into the snow when they tried to go further with it.

In spite of everything, or perhaps because of the poor logistics, the critical deficiency in their fight to and from the pole became food.

> The daily allowance of food for each man on the journey, as long as full rations were given, was to be as follows:

Pemmican	7.5 oz.
Emergency ration	1.5 oz.
Biscuit	16.0 oz.
Cheese or chocolate	2.0 oz.
Cocoa	0.7 oz.
Plasmon	1.0 oz.
Sugar	4.3 oz.
Quaker Oats	1.0 oz.
Total	34.0 oz.[14]

As it worked out, even eating three ponies and the corn intended for the ponies was insufficient; they did not have enough food and not enough carrying capacity.

They left on October 29, 1908, and on January 9, 1909, reached their furthest south: latitude 88° 23 minutes south, 162° east, less than 100 miles from the South Pole. The night before, Shackleton wrote, "I feel that this march must be our limit. We are so short of food, and at this high altitude, 11,600 ft., it is hard to keep any warmth in our bodies between the scanty meals."[15] Even before this, on December 31, Shackleton had calculated at latitude 86° 54 minutes south that they had only three weeks' food and two weeks' biscuits to do nearly 500 miles to and from the pole. He realized that this would be an impossible task. Averaging ten miles a day was excellent progress for them. On January 4 he wrote, "The end is in sight. We can only go for three more days at the most, for we are weakening rapidly."[16]

The return trip is a story of its own, full of descriptions of hunger, weakness, and disease, particularly dysentery. In his notes on the southern journey he wrote several pages on food:

> We brought back with us from the journey towards the Pole vivid memories of how it feels to be intensely, fiercely hungry. During the period from November 15, 1908, to February 23, 1909, we had but one full meal, and that was on Christmas Day. Even then we did not keep the sense of repletion for very long for within an hour or two it seemed to us that we were as hungry as ever. Our daily allowance of food would have been a small one for a city worker in a temperate climate, and in our case hunger was increased by the fact that we were performing vigorous physical labour in a very low temperature. We looked forward to each meal with keen anticipation, but when the food was in our hands it seemed to disappear without making us any the less ravenous. The evening meal at the end of ten hours' sledging used to take us a long time to prepare...We used to sit round the cooker waiting for our food, and at last the hoosh would be ready and would be ladled into the pannikins by the cook of the week. The scanty allowance of biscuit would be distributed and we would commence the meal. In a couple of minutes the hot food would be gone, and we would gnaw carefully round the sides of our biscuits, making them last as long as possible...If one of us dropped a crumb, the others would point it out, and the owner would wet his finger in his mouth and pick up the morsel. Not the smallest fragment was allowed to escape....We used 'turn backs' in order to ensure equitable division of the food.[17]

"Turn backs" was a procedure where one man would turn his back and then the others would point to one of the piles of food which had been divided into four equal parts, and the man with his back turned would say that this should be eaten by one of the four of them. The slightest difference in the amounts in each pile was enough to cause serious arguments.

How food occupied their thoughts, blinding them to the beauty around them, is seen in further notes:

> During the last weeks of the journey outwards, and the long march back, when our allowance of food had been reduced to twenty ounces per man a day, we really thought of little but food. The glory of the great mountains

that towered high on either side, the majesty of the enormous glacier up
which we travelled so painfully, did not appeal to our emotions to any great
extent. Man becomes very primitive when he is hungry and short of food,
and we learned to know what it is to be desperately hungry.[18]

During the first part of the trip the ponies had supplied them with additional food. They started eating the meat as soon as they killed the ponies,
an act that was done when a pony looked ill or was suffering. One of the
four ponies had been lost in a crevasse, a loss that Shackleton believed made
their journey that much less likely to succeed. With the ponies gone, they
then ate the ponies' corn. This worked out well when they merely mixed it
with water, but when it got very cold this mixture did not allow the corn to
absorb the water, a reaction that then occurred in the stomachs of the men,
causing them discomfort—a simple physical-chemical culinary problem, but
with harsh effects on starving men. Their hunger was relieved when they
discovered blood frozen into the snow from the killing of one of the ponies
on the way south. After digging it out and melting it, the coagulated blood
made a reviving meal for them.

After about 125 days away they made it back to base. Shackleton and
Wild had to go ahead during the last run because Marshall was extremely
ill, but within a few days Shackleton returned with a group to rescue Marshall,
and all recovered. If they had tried the last run for the pole, they surely
would have died of nutritional deficiencies and starvation.

In Shackleton's heart burned a fire to conquer Antarctica. After the South
Pole had been conquered by Amundsen and, in a way, by Scott with heroic
tales of his death, Shackleton chose a different heroic adventure, a
transantarctic crossing.[19] He named it "The Imperial Trans Antarctic Expedition," though support for the expedition—from the British Empire or any
other source—was not easy to muster for a variety of reasons. Attention was
focused on the coming war in Europe. Shackleton had to follow more or
less in the footsteps of the British hero, Scott, and money was very hard to
come by.

The expedition required a tremendous amount of preparation, and the
plan was extensive. It involved two ships and the establishment of two separate bases on opposite sides of the antarctic continent. The base for
Shackleton's own party was to be on the shore by the Weddell Sea, and the
second on the old spot of Ross Island. The object was for Shackleton to
make a 1,600-mile trek, crossing the continent via the pole using dogs and
mechanized transport. A party from Ross Island would go to the top of
Beardmore Glacier and leave depots of food and fuel along the way and at

the top. His first ship he named the *Endurance* for his own group, and the other was Douglas Mawson's old ship (Mawson having returned to Australia after his adventures in Antarctica), the *Aurora*. Little did Shackleton know at that time that *Endurance* would so greatly typify his subsequent exploits in overcoming the extensive difficulties of his trip. In the end, both groups endured the worst offered by Antarctica.

For the two ventures Shackleton equally divided his fifty-six man complement. The *Endurance*, with Shackleton and his group, took off from South Georgia on December 5, 1914. Shackleton's experienced six different very arduous and even hair-raising episodes during this expedition—and he never lost one of his twenty-eight-man contingent.[20]

The first episode was when the *Endurance* was beset and floated in the ice in the Weddell Sea, eventually foundering and sinking. The second was a nearly four months' encampment on the ocean ice, at a place Shackleton named Camp Patience because they had to wait patiently for the ice to break up in order to launch their small boats. The third was on April 13, when all twenty-eight men traveled 100 miles in three boats to Elephant Island. This was no mean event and required heavy work and good navigation, because if their point was missed by even a degree they could have been lost at sea. The fourth was reaching Elephant Island and setting up an encampment. The fifth was when Shackleton and four *five* others set off in one of the small boats and traveled 800 miles to the island of South Georgia to obtain help. And this was war time, with German raiders at sea. It was another sixteen days of heroic action by Shackleton. The sixth episode was the landing on South Georgia, followed by Shackleton's travel with two companions over the mountainous spine of South Georgia to a whaling station on the other side, a feat that was not accomplished by others until many years later—and then with much better equipment and on a much easier route.

Although at no time were any of Shackleton's men critically near starvation, many times food problems were serious, and because a lot of their efforts were on the high seas, potable water was also a problem. While at Camp Patience, the men supplemented their diet with fish, but fishing was not always successful. Good luck also played a part in their provisions. Though they were lucky as well as successful when a huge leopard seal was shot by one of the men, they were further rewarded upon discovering that its stomach contained large quantities of freshly consumed fish. This was a tasty addition to the diet, the only fish they had while there. Penguins and seals are not always plentiful because they follow the life cycle of the ocean

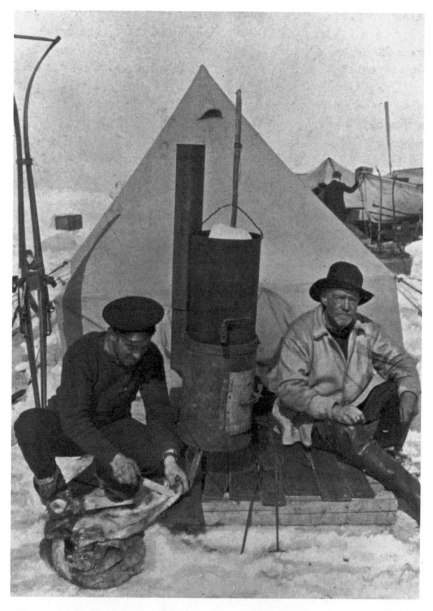

The stove at Shackleton's Patience Camp constructed out of old oil drums. Seal blubber and penguin skins were used as fuel. E. Shackleton, 1920

and move with the season. Although they had forty days' sledging rations, Shackleton kept these for their planned departure in the open boats. In the interim, food was severely rationed and was always on everybody's mind. He wrote:

> Another man searched for over an hour in the snow where he had dropped a piece of cheese some days before, in the hopes of finding a few crumbs...By this time blubber was a regular article of our diet—either raw, boiled or fried...As fuel is so scarce we have to resort to melting ice for drinking water in tins against our bodies.[21]

Shackleton was criticized for not setting up a stock of seal meat and penguins when they were plentiful for a while at Patience Camp. Roland Huntford thought that perhaps he did this in order to keep the morale of the men high, rather than have them think they would be imprisoned on top of the ice for too many months, waiting only to start a perilous journey in small boats.[22]

When they left Camp Patience the departure had to be quick because of the ice breaking. This caused them to have insufficient ice to melt for water, so the trip to Elephant Island was finished with thirsty men, whose lips were cracked and bodies dehydrated. In the whole venture, this voyage to Elephant Island has been dwarfed by the subsequent one to South Georgia. Both were dangerous, heroic, and well-administered voyages. At the encampment on Elephant Island twenty-three men waited for Shackleton's return, after he set off for South Georgia. On August 30, 1916, they were eating the last of their penguin and seal meat. The whole party had been collecting limpets and seaweed to eat with the stewed seal bones, which they had recovered from their pile of bones.[23] On that day, after four months, Shackleton returned to rescue them.

While these many complicated escapades of the *Endurance* expedition were going on, the other twenty-eight men from the *Aurora* had landed on Ross Island. The objective of the Ross Sea party, as it was called, was to lay depots from the Ross Sea to just north of the pole, supplying materials for Shackleton's hoped-for Trans Antarctic Expedition. They used the hut at Cape Evans where Scott had been during his second expedition. The depot group included the Reverend Arnold Spencer-Smith, Richards, Joyce, Hayward, Captain Mackintosh, and Earnest Wild. Unfortunately, the main notes were lost with the death of Captain Mackintosh on the return trip, when he and one other man were apparently drowned in the ocean. Still another died during the trip. Since Mackintosh kept the main notes, other diaries were relied upon for information about this unfortunate part of the

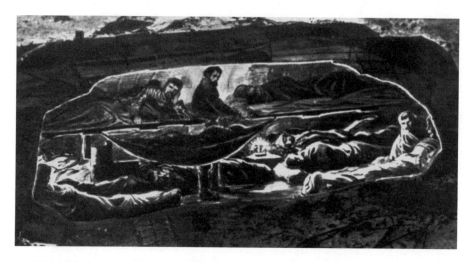

View of the interior of the hut on Elephant Island. Inside measurements were 18 feet x 9 feet x 5 feet at its highest point. Twenty-two men from Shackleton's main party lived in this hut for four and a half months. E. Shackleton, 1920

Trans Antarctic Expedition. Soon after their departure difficulties began to occur, the first of which was a breakdown of their motorized sledge. None of them were much good on skis, and as they went along they all came down with scurvy.[24]

Joyce, Wild, and Richards also had general symptoms: "Their joints became stiff and black in the rear." By February these men had been away from fresh food, and hence a source of vitamin C, for perhaps nearly five months. By February 29, on the way back, three of them were unable to go farther, having deteriorated to invalids. Two days later Spencer-Smith was dead. They arrived at Hut Point and Scott's old hut on March 18, having been away for 160 days and traveling 1,561 miles, all this time with but very little fresh meat from the animals they killed. There was plenty of food now, but they were still separated from the others at Cape Evans. Then, still another tragedy struck: Mackintosh and a companion were lost on the ice attempting to go to Cape Evans.

In spite of these many problems, they left ample food for Shackleton at the depots as planned. They had laid depots for the *Endurance* party that never got to the pole and over Beardmore Glacier to McMurdo Sound, and they had returned with half of the team dead. The time was near for an understanding of at least the broad concept of vitamins, and yet these explorers were greatly afflicted by scurvy and probably other vitamin deficiencies.

Notes

1. R. Huntford, *Scott and Amundsen* (London: Hodder and Stoughton, 1979); R. Huntford, *Shackleton* (NewYork: Random House (Ballantine Books), 1985); C. Ralling, *Shackleton* (London: British Broadcasting Corp., 1983); A. Lansing, *Endurance* (New York: McGraw-Hill Book Co., 1959); L. Bickel, *This Accursed Land* (Melbourne: Sun Books, 1978); C. Neider, *Edge of the World, Ross Island, Antarctica* (New York: Doubleday and Co., 1974; A. Cherry-Garrard, *The Worst Journey in the World* (London: Chatto and Windus Ltd., 1922).

2. Perhaps this led to his eventual disagreeable relationship with Shackleton. Scott was revered by those many people exclaiming "Great Scott!" In Shackleton's family circle this was changed to "Great Shack." But the public never adopted "Great Shack." Huntford, *Shackleton*, 3.

3. This ship was very different from Nansen's Norwegian ship, the *Fram*, which had been constructed to ride up on top of the ice if it were frozen in. See C. R. Markham, *The Land of Silence* (Cambridge: The University Press, 1921), 446.

4. Many of the men on board later became well known for their exploits in Antarctica on this trip and later ones. Geological features in the vicinity of Ross Island, McMurdo Sound, and on toward the South Pole were named after many of them. Standing high among those accompanying Scott were the two who did go with him toward the pole, Dr. Edmund Wilson and Shackleton. Many books and articles have been written about this expedition, unofficially called the *Discovery* expedition. R. F. Scott, *The Voyage of the Discovery* (London: John Murray, 1905).

5. R. F. Scott, *The Voyage of the Discovery*, 398–399.

6. Ibid., 400, 403, 404.

7. Ibid., 404–409.

8. Ibid., 320.

9. Ibid., 417.

10. Ibid., 485.

11. Ibid., 501.

12. E. Shackleton, *The Heart of the Antarctic* (Philadelphia: J. B. Lippincott, 1914); C. Ralling, *Shackleton* (London: British Broadcasting Corp., 1983), 1.

13. Ralling, *Shackleton*, 25.

14. Shackleton, *The Heart of the Antarctic*, 145.

15. Ibid., 209.

16. Ibid., 206.

17. Ibid., 229.

18. Ibid., 231.

19. E. Shackleton, *South* (New York: MacMillan, 1920), x.

20. Many books would be written on this expedition: Shackleton's own *South*, and those that were later written in detail, such as *Shackleton* by Huntford, *Shackleton* by Ralling, and *Endurance* by Lansing.

21. Shackleton, *South*, 112.

22. Huntford, *Shackleton*, 434.

23. Lansing, *Endurance*, 279.

24. Shackleton, *South*, 112.

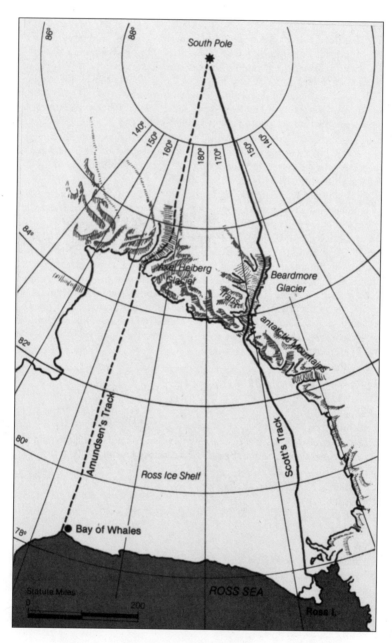

Scott's and Amundsen's south polar track. C. Neider

14

The Quest for the South Pole: Successes and Deaths

Amundsen, Scott, Shackleton, and Mawson were the 20th century's famous antarctic quartet. Of the four, Roald Amundsen and Captain Robert Falcon Scott probably differed the most in character and background: Scott, the British naval officer, and Amundsen, the Norwegian independent civilian and polar sailor. In early 1911 they were both in Antarctica preparing for their dash to the pole in the antarctic spring. Scott planned on several side expeditions and scientific observations; Amundsen's objective was to be first to reach the pole. They left within a few weeks of one another, both reaching the pole, but only Amundsen's final party made it out safely. Scott's five-man party perished.[1]

One could not have blamed ignorance for the dire outcome of his dash to the pole, for Robert Scott had made several trips to the south polar continent. Best known of these is the midwinter trip with Dr. Edward Wilson, Ashley Cherry-Garrard, and H. E. Bowers across Ross Island to the emperor penguin rookery at Cape Crozier to obtain some eggs. They had major difficulties on this trip, though not in the area of nutrition, but made it back safely.

At the beginning they had hoped to make this very cold journey an experiment on diets. As such, their plans initially included different diets for the three, but these ambitions had to be sacrificed under the harsh conditions. Wilson wrote,

> On July 6 Cherry felt the need for more food, and would have chosen fat, either butter or pemmican, had he not been experimenting on a large biscuit allowance. So he increased his biscuits to twelve a day, and found it did away to some extent with his desire for more food and fat. But he occasionally had heartburn, and had certainly felt the cold more than Bowers and I have, and has had more frostbite in hands, feet and face than we have.

I [Wilson] have altogether failed to eat anything approaching my allowance of 8 ozs. of butter a day. The most I have managed has been about 2 or 3 ozs.

Bowers has also found it impossible to eat his extra allowance of pemmican for lunch.

So yesterday—that is, a fortnight out—we decided that Cherry and I should both alter our diet, he to take 4 ozs. a day of my butter and I to take two of his biscuits, i.e. 4 ozs. in exchange.

This brought Cherry's diet and mine to the same. Bowers continued his diet, taking his extra pemmican when he felt it possible—but this became increasingly less frequent and all the way home he went without it.

Cherry's diet and mine was now, per diem:

Pemmican	2 ozs.
Biscuit	6 ozs.
Butter	4 ozs. (we rarely ate more than 2 ozs.)

Bowers' diet was now:

Pemmican	12 ozs.
Biscuit	16 ozs.
Extra pemmican	4 ozs. (rarely eaten).

Our daily routine was, for breakfast, to have first tea, then pemmican and biscuit; for lunch, tea and biscuit (and butter for Cherry and myself); for supper, hot water and pemmican and biscuit.

We none of us missed sugar or cocoa, or any of the other foods we have been used to on the sledge journey, and we all found we were amply satisfied on this diet. Cocoa would have been pleasanter at night than plain hot water, but the hot water with biscuit soaked in it was very good.[2]

One group that encountered some food and nutritional problems was the one Scott named the Northern Party. This party, consisting of seven men under the leadership of Lt. Commander V. L. A. Campbell, eventually spent nearly a year in a cave dug out of the ice.[3] The group consisted of navy men except for a civilian geologist and meteorologist, Raymond Priestley.[4] In February of 1911 they were dropped by the ship *Terra Nova* for exploration 200 miles north of McMurdo Sound. But the ship was unable to return and so they found themselves unintentionally, and unexpectedly, abandoned—an accident that led to one of the most incredible adventures in polar history.

Campbell's Northern Party had taken ashore only enough provisions for a six-week sledge journey, plus an emergency food ration for two weeks. Campbell gave close attention to their food:

For some days we have been preparing in every way possible for the winter, and our position may be summed up as follows: We landed, besides our sledging rations, six boxes of biscuits with 45 lbs. in each box. The sledging biscuits were finished March 1, and of the others we have to keep two boxes intact for our journey down the coast.

We have also enough cocoa to give us a mug of very thin cocoa five nights of the week; enough tea for a mug of equally thin tea once a week; and the remaining day we must reboil the tea leaves or drink hot water solus. Our only luxuries are a very small amount of chocolate and sugar, sufficient to give us a stick of chocolate every Saturday and every other Wednesday, and eight lumps of sugar every Sunday. A bag of raisins we are keeping to allow twenty-five raisins per man on birthdays and red-letter days, and I can see that one of Priestley's difficulties in the future is going to be preventing each man from having a birthday once a month. We have decided to open up neither the chocolate not the sugar till we are settled in our winter quarters, and, at present, breakfast and supper each consist of a mug of weak seal hoosh and one of weak cocoa, with one biscuit.[5]

They also carried several cases of oxtail bouillon. On February 23, still waiting for the ship, they decided to ration their food and establish quarters in a cave on an island, three miles long by half a mile broad, a mile or so off the continent.

By a little over a month and a half later, their rations and cooking had changed from their original plans. On April 5:

Our rations at this time were as follows: Breakfast, 1 mug of penguin and seal hoosh and 1 biscuit. Supper one and a half mugs of seal, one biscuit and three quarters of a pint of thin cocoa, tea, or hot water. We were always hungry on this, and to swell the hoosh we used occasionally to try putting in seaweed, but most of it had deteriorated owing to the heat of the sun and the attentions of the penguins.

The cocoa we could only afford to have five days a week and then very thin, but as we had a little tea we had weak tea on Sunday and reboiled the leaves for Monday. As already stated we had a little chocolate (two ounces per man a week), and eight lumps of sugar every Sunday. Our tobacco soon ran out, even with the most rigid economy, and we were reduced to smoking the much-boiled tea and wood shavings—a poor substitute. About the middle of this month we found we were getting through our seal meat too fast, so had to come down to half the above ration, and it was not until the middle of July, when we got some more seals, that we were able to go back to the old ration.

These is no doubt that during this period we were all miserably hungry, even directly after meals. Towards the end of June we had to cut down still more, and have only one biscuit per day, and after July to stop the biscuit ration altogether until September, when we started one biscuit a day again. By this means we were able to save enough biscuits for a month at half ration for our journey down the coast. I am sure seals have never been so

thoroughly eaten as ours were. There was absolutely no waste. The brain
was our greatest luxury; then the liver, kidneys, and heart, which we used to
save for Sundays. The bones, after we had picked all the meat off them, we
put on one side, so that if the worst came to the worst we could pound them
up for soup. The best of the undercuts was saved for sledging. After our
experience in March, when we got thirty-nine fish out of a seals stomach,
we always cut them open directly (after) we killed them in the hope of
finding more, but we never again found anything fit to eat. One of our
greatest troubles was a lack of variety in the flavouring of our meals. Two
attempts were made by Levick to relieve this want from the medicine chest,
but both were failures. Once we dissolved several ginger tabloids in the
hoosh without any effect at all, and on the historic occasion when we used
a mustard plaster, there was a general decision that the correct term would
have been linseed plaster, as the mustard could not be tasted at all and the
flavour of linseed was most distinct.[6]

The meal routine was something like this: they made a hoosh (thick soup
or stew) of whatever they had and then they opened their biscuit box. They
would put out the biscuits on the sugar box and give equal portions to each
man. They obtained an occasional seal or penguin. When in the spring they
were able to kill four emperor penguins, this gave them about 100 pounds
of meat which was a boon to their diet. Quoting from Priestley:

> One great discovery in the edible line was the use of ice soaked in seal's
> blood for our hooshes (ice had to be melted for water). When the seal was
> butchered the hot blood melted down into the ice and the pool thus formed
> froze solid a few hours later. Then one of us would go down with a pick and
> shovel and a sack and dig up this mixture of blood and ice and carry it into
> the cave. Part of this was then boiled up in the hoosh and this made a gravy
> in which it was possible to stand a spoon upright. From the savings of their
> initial rations it was possible for some time to serve out twelve lumps of
> sugar to each man every Sunday, plus 1 1/2 ounces of chocolate every Sat-
> urday and every alternate Wednesday two small cans of cocoa for the group,
> and finally 25 individual raisins for the last day of each month. Five days of
> each week the cook threw into a pot full of boiling water three teaspoons of
> cocoa and this just sufficed to disguise the flavor of the blubber. On Sunday
> three teaspoons of tea performed the same. On Monday the same tea leaves
> were boiled in the water. Finally, the tea leaves were dried and ground up
> with wood shavings and used for tobacco. Once every three days we had
> oxal hoosh (bouillon), and these mornings were very looked forward to with
> keen anticipation.[7]

In preparation for the march south to Scott's main camp, they unearthed
the pemmican that they had been saving for this effort. It was then that the
pemmican was truly appreciated by Priestley: "I have picked up delicacies at
depots along a long line of march and other treats, but on such an occasion

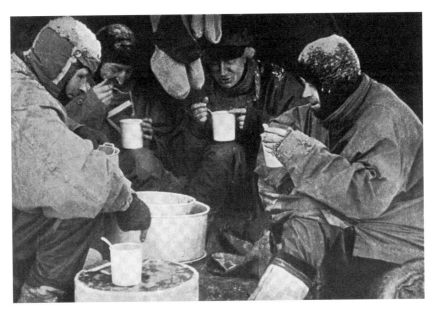

A meal on Scott's march. From H. Ponting, *The Great White South*, 1922

I would willingly have given these luxuries for half the weight of the regulation pemmican."[8]

Their sledging ration per man was:

2 pannikins of meat	1 stick of chocolate
3/4 pannikin of blubber	8 lumps of sugar
1 pannikin of cocoa	A little pemmican
3 biscuits[9]	

They left on October 1. On the way south they encountered a small depot at Cape Roberts which alleviated their hunger, but their mouths became terribly sore from eating some of this cached food. Priestley commented, "This, I suppose, had to do with the biscuit eating but very likely, as I now reflect on it, it was certainly due in part to the fact that we were close to outright scurvy."[10] When they arrived at Cape Evans on November 7, they were badly undernourished. "We weighed on our arrival at the hut and found ourselves much below normal. We certainly had discovered symptoms of edema, which is a marked symptom of scurvy.... I find our party is not so fit as I thought. Most of us have developed swollen ankles and legs (edema), and when the flesh is pressed in the holes remain there."[11]

On half or even quarter rations for some periods, and with some meat from penguins and seals, they made it, one of the last expeditions to be isolated with such limited faculties for so long, eight and one half months. Half starved, filthy, greasy and blackened from the soot of burning blubber in their ice cave, thin and scorbutic, they were an unwholesome sight. The late Sir Charles Wright, a geologist, told me that when he saw them at the hut at Cape Evans: "They looked like creatures who had crawled up from the depths of the earth."[12]

While the northern party under Campbell was fighting for their lives, the two great south-polar explorers, Robert Falcon Scott and Roald Amundsen, were on their way to the South Pole.

Robert Scott was born in England in 1868. Coming from a long line of British naval officers, he was thirteen years old when he became a cadet in training. By age twenty-one he was a lieutenant and, after several assignments and completing training in torpedoes, in 1893 he was given command of a torpedo boat. He ran his first assignment aground, an incident abhorred by all young British naval officers because such a black mark on their records would hinder their advancement through normal peacetime channels. The accident has been thought to be the reason he sought fame and promotion through polar exploration, for the lists of higher ranking officers who had been promoted over others after completing polar explorations showed Scott that this different route to advancement could succeed. Besides, being a polar explorer was a lot more adventurous than being a torpedo officer. Thus, he had found his career. Working all angles, in 1901 he was put in command of his first antarctic expedition on the *Discovery*. As we have seen, all was done properly, according to navy rules, regulations, and customs, as should have been expected.[13]

On his next, and final, antarctic expedition, Scott was still the dedicated naval officer. In his book, Lt. Evans, who had hoped until the last minute to be a member of the final polar party, summarized the accepted beliefs on the philosophy underlying Scott's expedition: "The main object of our expedition was to reach the South Pole and secure for the British nation the honour of that achievement, but the attainment of the Pole was far from being the only object in view, for Scott intended to extend his former discoveries and bring back a rich harvest of scientific results."[14]

Roald Amundsen, born in Norway in 1872, also was from a family with a seafaring heritage, but that of a Norwegian merchant marine life rather than a British naval one. Learning to ski came with learning to walk. As a young teenager, Amundsen was already reading stories of the polar explorers, but his father soon sent him off to medical school, an educational experience he found boring. He wanted to be a sailor and became one, eventually getting his master's papers. Then the polar spirit engulfed him. Soon he was in Antarctica on the Belgian ship, the *Belgica*, and shortly afterward engaged in his famous northwest passage on the *Gjoa*. Acquiring the friendship and approval of Nansen, he obtained the use of the *Fram* and began to develop plans for the South Pole. Amundsen was not of the British heroic cult like Scott, nor was he much interested in science for the sake of science. For him, science and technology were only tools for the everyday needs of the exploration. He wanted to be first.

Just a few years after his valiant but unsuccessful attempt to reach the pole, Scott set about organizing another extensive south polar expedition. Although the main object was to be the first to reach the South Pole, scientific observations were to be included. Back he went to McMurdo Sound, this time to Cape Evans rather than to Hut Point, and he wintered over there to get ready for his dash the coming antarctic spring. He had with him his old friend and former Antarctic colleague, Dr. Edward Wilson. He put his faith in British naval zeal. Motor sledges and ponies rather than polar dogs were to do the main hauling, and the men were still outfitted with the old tight-fitting clothing with a separate hat. These were not minor points: The motor sledges were untried, ponies had to have fodder, and even British zeal could not compensate for the poor knowledge of human nutrition at the time.

Although the year 1911 was probably a ripe one for attempting to reach the pole, the role of vitamins in preventing many diseases had not yet been shown—the explorers could have only faith in Lind's now very old recommendations on the one hand, and the near-opposite beliefs like ptomaine causations related to scurvy on the other. And little was realized as to deficiencies in B vitamins. Only common sense in relying on the previous experiences and reports could be invoked. So Scott was still back at the point of his previous *Discovery* expedition, with perhaps a few more concerns. While the group was making preparations at Cape Evans, Sir Ralph Atkinson gave a lecture to the men that summarized what Scott believed at that time (August 18, 1911):

Atkinson lectured on 'Scurvy' last night. He spoke clearly and slowly, but the disease is anything but precise. He gave a little summary of its history afloat and the remedies long in use in the Navy.

He described the symptoms with some detail. Mental depression, debility, syncope, petechia, livid patches, spongy gums, lesions, swellings, and so on to things that are worse. He passed to some of the theories held and remedies tried in accordance with them. Ralph came nearest to the truth in discovering decrease of chlorine and alkalinity of urine. Sir Almroth Wright has hit the truth, he thinks, in finding increased acidity of blood—acid intoxication—by methods only possible in recent years.

This acid condition is due to two salts, sodium hydrogen carbonate and sodium hydrogen phosphate; these cause the symptoms observed and infiltration of fat in organs, leading to feebleness of heart action. The method of securing and testing serum of patient was described (titration, a colorimetric method of measuring the percentage of substances in solution), and the test by litmus paper of normal or super-normal solution. In this test the ordinary healthy man shows normal 30 to 50: the scurvy patient normal 90.

Lactate of sodium increases alkalinity of blood, but only within narrow limits, and is the only chemical remedy suggested.

So far for diagnosis, but it does not bring us much closer to the cause, preventives, or remedies. Practically we are much as we were before, but the lecturer proceeded to deal with the practical side.

In brief, he holds the first cause to be tainted food, but secondary or contributory causes may be even more potent in developing the disease, damp, cold, over-exertion, bad air, bad light, in fact any condition exceptional to normal healthy existence. Remedies are merely to change these conditions for the better. Dietetically, fresh vegetables are the best curatives— the lecturer was doubtful of fresh meat, but admitted its possibility in Polar climate; lime juice only useful if regularly taken. He discussed lightly the relative values of vegetable stuffs, doubtful of those containing abundance of phosphates such as lentils. He touched theory again in continuing the cause of acidity to bacterial action—and the possibility of infection in epidemic form. Wilson is evidently slow to accept the 'acid intoxication' theory; his attitude is rather 'non proven.' His remarks were extremely sound and practical as usual. He proved the value of fresh meat in Polar regions.

Scurvy seems very far away from us this time; yet after our *Discovery* experience, one feels that no trouble can be too great or no precaution too small to be adopted to keep it at bay. Therefore such an evening as last was well spent.

It is certain we shall not have the disease here, but one cannot forsee equally certain avoidance in the southern journey to come. All one can do is to take every possible precaution.[15]

On October 24 two motor sledges started ahead of Scott's main group, hauling material, but they didn't get very far because both broke down and had to be abandoned. Scott himself left on November 1 with eight ponies, each with a sled. Dogs were used, following later, but were not to be taken to the pole. Even as early as November 7 Scott was tent bound in a blizzard.

Travel was difficult. Ponies sank in the snow, but even more important, the ponies suffered terribly at night. When they would sweat, ice would form on their bodies as they stood. Though dogs did not suffer from the harsh conditions, Scott did not appreciate their advantage over ponies. He disowned the idea that dogs could eat dogs, and especially that men could eat dogs. When the final return party that had helped bring and set up depots left, Scott made the fateful decision to increase his group going to the pole from four to five, even though the food had been proportioned out for four men and tenting was provided for only four. In addition, the added man had no skis because of an earlier decision Scott had made that the last return party would not take skis. At this point they were all man-hauling. Yet for a brief time all seemed well. Just three days later was Christmas with such a plentiful supper that Scott wrote they had eaten too much:

> I must write a word of our supper last night. We had four courses. The first, pemmican, full whack, with slices of horse meat flavoured with onion and curry powder and thickened with biscuits; then an arrowroot, cocoa and biscuit hoosh sweetened; then a plum-pudding; then cocoa with raisins, and finally desert of caramels and ginger. After the feast it was difficult to move. Wilson and I couldn't finish our plates of plum-pudding. We have all slept splendidly and feel thoroughly warm—such is the effect of full feeding.[16]

The group arrived at the pole exhausted. Then came the terrible blow to their morale: Amundsen had been there before them. Their fateful return started on January 25. They were Scott, Dr. Wilson, Captain Lawrence E. G. Oates, Lt. Henry R. Bowers, and Seaman Edgar Evans (ages: Scott, 43; Wilson, 39; Oates, 32; Bowers, 28; Evans, 37). Now they had to man-haul from the pole back to Hut Point, a distance of around 800 miles. Soon they were frequently stalled by very bad weather, exhausted and barely making each depot before running out of food, even when on partial rations. By February 14, they were proceeding poorly:

> There is no getting away from the fact that we are not pulling strong. Probably none of us: Wilson's leg still troubles him and he doesn't like to trust himself on ski; but the worst case is Evans, who is giving us serious anxiety. This morning he suddenly disclosed a huge blister on his foot. It delayed us on the march, when he had to have his crampon readjusted. Sometimes I fear he is going from bad to worse, but I trust he will pick up again when we come to steady work on ski like this afternoon. He is hungry and so is Wilson. We can't risk opening our food again, and as cook at present I am serving something under full allowance. We are inclined to get slack and slow with our camping arrangements, and small delays increase. I

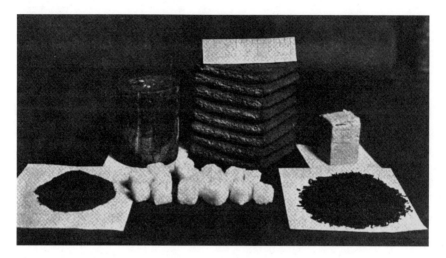

The sledging ration of Scott's party for one man for one day. A. F. Rogers, 1974

have talked of the matter tonight and hope for improvement. We cannot do distance without the hours. The next depot some thirty miles away and nearly 3 days food in hand.[17]

Then came two terrible fatalities. The first was the death of Seaman Edgar Evans, a large man, who complained that he received the same ration as the rest of them but his body required more. In retrospect, one can say that his complaints were well founded. However, sometime earlier he had had an accident to his head, which, at the time, was thought to be part of the cause of his infirmity. Finally he lagged behind the group, collapsed off the trail, and died. Perhaps if Scott had been able to read what Peary wrote a few years later, Seaman Evans might not have been selected for the party:

> Small, wiry men have a great advantage over large ones in polar work. The latter require more material for their clothing, and usually eat more than the former. Large men take up more space than small ones, necessitating the building of larger snow igloos when on the march, or the carrying of larger tents than would be needed for a party made up of small men. Every pound in weight beyond the maximum requirement tends to lessen a man's agility; in fact, renders him clumsy and more apt to break his equipment. For instance, if a large man on snow-shoes stumbles, a sudden lunge to save himself more often than not results in a broken snow-shoe.[18]

By March 5 they still had a long way to go, but with a favorable wind they still made nine miles. Yet, Scott knew things were bad:

Lunch—Regret to say going from bad to worse. We got a slant of wind yesterday afternoon, and going on five hours we converted our wretched morning run of three and a half miles to something over nine. We went to bed on a cup of cocoa and pemmican solid with the chill off.

The result is telling on all, but mainly on Oates, whose feet are in a wretched condition. One swelled up tremendously last night and he is very lame this morning. We started march on tea and pemmican as last night— we pretend to prefer the pemmican this way.[19]

Oates indeed had started failing rapidly, particularly with very bad feet; he was the next fatality. One morning when he left the tent all knew where he was going—to walk out and never return.[20] By this time all three of the others also were suffering in various ways, particularly Dr. Wilson. On Wednesday, March 21, they stopped. Scott wrote:

Got within 11 miles of One Ton Depot on Monday night; had to lay up all day yesterday in severe blizzard. Today forlorn hope. Wilson and Bowers going to depot for fuel. March 22 and 23. Blizzard bad as ever—Wilson and Bowers unable to start—tomorrow last chance—no fuel and only one or two of food left—must be near the end. Have decided it shall be natural—we shall march for the depot with or without our effects and die in our tracks. (March 29.) Since the 21st we have had a continuous gale from W.S.W and S.W. We had fuel to make two cups of tea apiece and bare food for two days on the 20th. Every day we have been ready to start for our depot 11 miles away, but outside the door of the tent it remains a scene of whirling drift. I do not think we can hope for any better things now. We shall stick it out to the end, but we are getting weaker, of course, and the end cannot be far. It seems a pity but I do not think I can write more. R. Scott. Last entry. For God's sake, look after our people.[21]

Scott also left a message to the public to explain the reasons for the tragedy:

1) The loss of pony transport in March 1911 obliged me to start later than I had intended and obliged the limits of stuff transported to be narrowed.

2) The weather throughout the outward journey and especially the long gale in 83° south stopped us.

3) The soft snow and lower reaches of glacier again reduced the pace.[22]

Scott went on to say he thought they had enough food and depots properly placed. He believed that Edgar Evans had received a concussion of the brain and that he died a natural death.

There have been many analyses of the Scott expedition and the reasons why they did not make it back. The weak link in the end was the food and nutrition. This failure was not entirely Scott's fault, because the knowledge of nutrition at that time was insufficient to formulate the diet properly. From comments made in various places, it is apparent that malnutrition occurred, and especially with Seaman Evans, scurvy is suspected.

If poor nutrition was the foremost problem, other factors still played a role. Scott's selection of ponies over dogs as the main animal-hauling power was incorrect. He had improperly contained and insufficient fuel; the bungs on the cans were such that the fuel was lost by vaporization. A fourth inadequacy was the clothing and sleeping bags; they were not like those of the Eskimo.

A fifth and possible crucial deficiency was Scott's decision to add a man, increasing the team to the pole from four to five. Scott may have done this in order to insure that each branch of the British armed forces was represented in the polar team. As a result, the fifth man did not have skis, and the rations and tent accommodations that were planned for four had to be shared by five. There would have been better traveling if Scott had followed Peary's recommendation, written in 1890, that "every increase in the party, beyond the number absolutely essential, [increases] an element of danger and failure."[23]

Apsley Cherry-Garrard in his beautiful book, *The Worst Journey in the World*, stated "I have always had a doubt whether the weather conditions were sufficient to cause the tragedy."[24] He goes on to indicate that even back when he wrote his book, it could be shown that there were insufficient calories:

> Of course the whole business simply bristles with 'ifs': if Scott had taken dogs and succeeded in getting them up the Beardmore: if we had not lost those ponies on the depot journey: if the dogs had not been taken so far and the One Ton Depot had been laid: if a pony and an extra oil had been depoted on the barrier: if a four-man party had been taken to the Pole: if I had disobeyed my instructions and gone on for One Ton, killing dogs as necessary: or even if I had just gone on a few miles and left some food and fuel under a flag upon a carrion: if they had been first at the Pole: if it had been any other season but that....[25]

Cherry-Garrard was deeply affected by a failed rescue attempt that he and one other man made with dogs to One Ton Depot at the time Scott was still traveling. Scott had left orders that the dogs were not to be pushed hard, and in addition, One Ton Depot had not had dog food left there because of transportation and weather problems. So Cherry-Garrard and his companion, after waiting a few days, returned to Hut Point. Many think he spent his life believing he could have saved Scott if he had gone farther

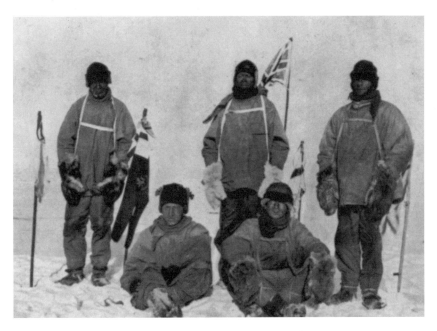

Scott's party at the South Pole, from left to right: Capt. Oates, Lieut. Bowers,
Capt. Scott, Dr. Wilson, and P. O. Evans. L. Huxley, 1913

than One Ton, killing dogs as needed, but this would have been against
Scott's original order (remember that Scott ended just eleven miles from
One Ton).

The Norwegian expedition was profoundly different in planning,
execution, and outcome. After the 1908 announcement of Cook's discovery
of the North Pole and then Peary's expedition there in 1909, Amundsen
had begun to think of the South Pole. The north may have been won, but
the south was open to his attack. His plans to attain the South Pole were
accurately and extensively made, but that he was going there was kept a
secret. This was done because his financial support and political support
(particularly from Nansen) was for achieving the North Pole by sailing up
through the Bering Sea. It was only while the competitor he feared so much,
Scott, was actually in New Zealand making final plans for the South Pole
that Amundsen notified Scott that he was actually en route.

Amundsen felt no compunction:

> Nor did I feel any great scruples with regards to the other Antarctic expedi-
> tions that were being planned at the time. I knew I should be able to inform

Captain Scott the extension of my plans before he left civilization and therefore a few months sooner or later could be of no great importance. Scott's
plan and equipment were so widely different from my own that I regarded
the telegram which I sent him later, with the information that we were
bound for the Antarctic regions, rather as a mark of courtesy than as a communication which might cause him to alter his program in the slightest
degree. The British expedition was designed entirely for scientific research.
The Pole was only a side issue, whereas in my extended plan it was the main
object. On this little detour science would have to look after itself; but of
course I knew very well we could not reach the Pole by the route I had
determined to take without enriching in a considerable degree several
branches of science.[26]

He decided on the Bay of Whales for a base, which was the other side of
Ross Island and sixty miles closer to the pole—120 miles closer round trip.
Food and supplies were of major importance. He analyzed Shackleton's trip
and concluded that larger depots were needed along the way. Amundsen's
idea that fresh meat prevented scurvy was a critical point. However, for
energy on these long trips he needed pemmican. A perhaps fortunate set-
back occurred when Armour of Chicago cancelled their promise to give
free pemmican.[27] From Amundsen's polar work he knew that straight heavy
food might cause some problems for some men from stomach ailments,
constipation, and diarrhea, all of which could cause great difficulties on a
polar trail. So he had specially prepared pemmican made, first adding
vegetables and later oatmeal for fiber.

Amundsen arrived at the Bay of Whales in January 1911. Only slightly
prior to that time did Scott receive the wire that Amundsen was proceeding
to the South Pole. Nansen also was notified. The *Fram* was at the edge of
the ice, and a skillfully designed hut was set up on January 27. Two hundred
seals and the same number of penguins were killed and frozen for food.
When the expedition members laid the depots at good marches, there was
plenty of food at each place. They went to 82° south for the last depot, 400
miles from the South Pole.

At Framheim (the name of his base) the food was excellently cooked.
Served daily twice for lunch and supper, the main food was fresh or deep-
frozen seal. The men also got berry preserves. Amundsen directed that the
seal meat be undercooked, thereby saving much of the vitamin C. All through
the subsequent winter Amundsen's group was storing up vitamin C,
vitamin D, and probably most all the vitamin B complex. They had whole
meal bread fortified with wheat germ and leavened with fresh yeast (both
later to be known as good sources of B vitamins). This was what healthy and

rugged Norwegians ate, something that Amundsen knew and that was his basis for sledding provisions:

> I have never considered it necessary to take a whole grocery shop with me when sledding; the food should be simple and nourishing and that is enough—a rich and varied menu is for people who have no work to do. Besides pemmican, we had biscuits, milk powder and chocolate. The biscuits were a present from a well-known Norwegian factory and did all honors to their origin. They were specially baked for us and made of oatmeal with the addition of dried milk and a little sugar; they were extremely nourishing and pleasant to the taste; thanks to efficient packing they kept fresh and crisp all the day. These biscuits formed a great part of our daily diet and undoubtedly contributed in no small degree to the successful result. Milk powder is a comparatively new commodity with us but it deserves to be better known. It came from the District of Jaederen. Neither heat nor cold, dryness or wet could hurt it; we had large quantities of it lying out in small thin linen bags in every possible state of the weather: the powder was as good the last day as the first. We also took dried milk from a firm in Wisconsin; this milk had an addition of malt and sugar, and was, in my opinion, excellent; it also kept good the whole time. The chocolate came from a world-renowned firm and was beyond all praise. The whole supply was a very acceptable gift....We are bringing all the purveyors of our sledging samples of their goods that have made the journey to the South Pole and back in gratitude for the kind assistance they afforded us.[28]

Amundsen had provisioned so prudently that he actually had spare food to return as souvenirs to the temperate zone. On October 20 they left Framheim for the pole. Though the party originally had been planned to consist of eight, Amundsen reduced it to five. Now there was an even more adequate supply of food deposited along the way. At the last phase of his trek towards the pole, Scott had increased his group from four to five; this decision too contrasted with Amundsen's dropping from eight to five. At 82° south, 420 miles to the pole, he had supplies for 100 days, until February 6, but he hoped to return to Framheim by January 31. He had indeed a big margin of safety, because these estimates did not include the depot at 82° plus a previous depot, so if he missed all the depots on return his supplies were adequate enough so that he could still make it with a week to spare. The party slaughtered dogs en route and fed them to the remaining dogs, as well as to themselves, and they also placed extra carcasses at depots for their return. By this time, the men even savored the idea of eating fresh dog cutlets:

> But the thought of the fresh dog cutlets that awaited us when we got to the top made our mouths water. In the course of time we had so habituated

ourselves to the idea of the approaching slaughter of dogs that this event did not appear to us so horrible as it would otherwise have done.[29]

The dog cutlets appeared to be a welcome addition to the general ration, although that was well organized.

On restocking their provisions they made their supplies in such a form that they could count them instead of weighing them:

> Our pemmican was in rations of one-half kilogram (1 pound 1-1/2 ounces). The chocolate was divided into small pieces, as chocolate always is, so that we knew what each piece weighed. Our milk-powder was put up in bags of 10-1/2 ounces—just enough for a meal. Our biscuits possessed the same property—they could be counted, but this was a tedious business, as they were rather small. On this occasion we had to count 6,000 biscuits. Our provisions consisted of only these four kinds, and the combinations turned out right enough. We did not suffer from a craving either for fat or sugar, though the want of these substances is very commonly felt on such journeys as ours. In our biscuits we had an excellent product, consisting of oatmeal, sugar, and dried milk. Sweetmeats, jam, fruit, cheese, etc., we had left behind at Framheim.[30]

At 88° 23 minutes, ninety miles from the pole, Amundsen carefully laid the depot that would be the first stop on the way out. At this point he had seventeen dogs (one ran away). They arrived at the pole on December 16. After making careful measurements, leaving a tent and a note for Scott, they were soon headed back towards the north. Finally, after the half-way point, there were frequent depots. The rations were increased by 500 calories (from maybe 4500 to 5000). On reaching the main depot at 85° 5 minutes south on January 6, they found everything in order, with more supplies than they needed:

> We reached the depot, and found everything in order. The heat here must have been very powerful; our lofty, solid depot was melted by the sun into a rather low mound of snow. The pemmican rations that had been exposed to the direct action of the sun's rays had assumed the strangest forms, and, of course, they had become rancid. We got the sledges ready at once, taking all the provisions out of the depot and loading them. We left behind some of the old clothes we had been wearing all the way from here to the Pole and back. When we had completed all this repacking and had everything ready, two of us went over to Mount Betty, and collected as many different speci-mens of rock as we could lay our hands on. At the same time we built a great cairn, and left there a can of 17 litres of paraffin, two packets of matches—containing twenty boxes—and an account of our expedition. Possibly someone may find a use for these things in the future.[31]

Not only did they have plenty of rations, they had frozen seal meat as well:

> On our way southward we had taken a good deal of seal meat and had divided it among the depots we built on the Barrier in such a way that we were now able to eat fresh meat every day. This had not been done without an object; if we should be visited by scurvy, this fresh meat would be invaluable. As we were—sound and healthy as we had never been before—the seal-beef was a pleasant distraction in our menu, nothing more.[32]

At 82° south they had pemmican and seal steaks, with chocolate pudding for dessert. Three dogs had died, and they had to kill one, reducing them to thirteen. When the dead ones were fed to the remaining thirteen, they seemed to liven up. The dogs were put on double rations of pemmican, seal meat, biscuits, and even chocolate later on. On reaching the big depot at 80° south they considered they were back. Here again they left a depot well supplied: "The depot at 80° south is still large, well supplied and well marked, so it is not impossible that it may be found useful later."[33]

The last leg, from 80° south to Framheim, was easily done. On January 25, they returned with a dozen dogs, as originally planned, and with men and dogs all in good shape, and in ninety-nine days (Scott's time was more than 140 days).

How could two men with such closely similar feelings about polar discoveries and with such fervor and assiduous attention to planning their explorations produce expeditions so different in outcome? This has been debated many times, but as already noted, their backgrounds and personalities were very different—Scott, the British naval officer; Amundsen, the Norwegian civilian sailor—and these differences are accepted by many historians as being responsible for the differences in their polar operations. Certainly how they went about planning their attacks and getting to the pole were very different. At their main bases things also were very different. Amundsen kept everyone busy at communal living. Following naval custom, Scott separated the officers and the scientists from the rest of the group by means of a partition. With Amundsen everybody worked in repairing, building, packing, and other preparations for the expedition to the pole. With Scott this was done mainly by navy ratings. Amundsen literally forced his people to eat nearly raw seal meat, while Scott deferred for a while, and even then the meat was cooked more to English customs.

Much has been said about dogs, ponies, and motor sledges. Amundsen's dog sledging to the pole and back stands in sharp contrast to Scott's extensive man-hauling. Reducing his polar party from eight to five (due to personnel considerations) was a fortunate development for Amundsen and certainly helped him considerably, since he had planned his depots for eight. In contrast, Scott's increase of his party from four to five was probably disastrous, since food was present and distributed for only four. Scott's clothing was more like British sportsmen's ski outfits, which had separate head gear, while Amundsen had two types, one an Eskimo fur jacket and the other a Norwegian-type anorak with an attached fur around the face.

In the end, though, it was the nutritional deficiencies that made the difference. According to Cherry-Garrard:

> Undoubtedly the low temperatures caused their death, inasmuch as they would have lived had the temperatures remained high. But Evans would not have lived: he died before the low temperatures occurred. What killed Evans? And why did the other men weaken as they did, though they were eating full rations and more? Weaken so much that in the end they starved to death?
>
> I have always had a doubt whether the weather conditions were sufficient to cause the tragedy. These men on full rations were supposed to be eating food of sufficient value to enable them to do the work they were doing, under the conditions which they actually met until the end of February, without loss of strength. They had more than their full rations, but the conditions in March were much worse than they imagined to be possible: when three survivors out of the five pitched their Last Camp they were in a terrible state. After the war I found that Atkinson had come to wonder much as I, but he had gone farther, for he had the values of our rations worked out by a chemical expert according to the latest knowledge and standards. I may add that, being in command after Scott's death, he increased the ration for the next year's sledging, so I suppose he had already come to the conclusion that the previous ration was not sufficient.[34]

As to Chief Petty Officer Evans' illness and eventual death, A. F. Rogers has concluded that early scurvy was the cause of his death. In his article Rogers discussed three possibilities.[35] The first was a general infection, which he thinks unlikely from Wilson's comments. Second, he thought that maybe Evans was deficient in vitamins and also had a cerebral form of beriberi, but he does not think this is likely. Finally, he stated, "The third and most likely explanation is that Evans had early scurvy with the result that a minor head injury caused an intercranial hemorrhage." But no information was available on the appearance of the bodies of the three in that deathly frozen tent. Certainly they all three probably had scurvy, as well as some deficiencies of B vitamins and definitely a calorie deficiency.

Not only did Scott's final party end in their tragic nutritional condition, but his last supporting party, on their return, likewise encountered scurvy and other serious deficiencies in nutrition.[36] The last supporting party had almost as long a trek back, having started their return only 148 miles from the pole.[37] There were only three, Lt. Edward Evans (no relation to Edgar), Thomas Crean, and William Lashley, because Scott had taken one of their originally planned four with him to the pole. This meant they had to spend extra time each day rearranging the equipment and supplies originally planned for four. Crevasses, mountains, snow variations (wetness), and blizzards dogged them. Slowly Lt. Evans began to deteriorate, finally developing scurvy when they had been out for ninety-one days. He had to be carried the last ten days of the trip and was reported to have almost died.

A look at Scott's rations does not add to its appeal for us today, nor does it tell us its nutritional value. Rogers' analysis of Scott's diet is given in table 14.1 (page 160).[38] Although these figures are estimates, they indicate deplorable nutrition. Of course, as already stated, much of this was unavoidable because of the ignorance about vitamins at that time. But the calorie deficiency should not have occurred. In addition, Amundsen shored up his men with good nutrition before departure and, knowingly or not, supplied them with a more nutritious diet, particularly for vitamins, while en route to the pole. Also, of course, his requirements were much less because he was much faster and did not use the energy for exhaustive man-hauling. On much of the way to the pole, Amundsen's party was even pulled on their skis by their dogs. In an in-depth summary of the relationship between the nutrition and energy requirements of both expeditions, H. E. Lewis compared both the men and dogs.[39] Dogs need about the same amount of energy for activity, but they do better hauling. Probably of equal importance, dogs synthesize their own vitamin C, helping both the dogs and the men who eat them.

Huntford has further summarized the differences in diet.

Scott's sledging ration from the Beardmore Glacier onwards, per man and day, was 20 gm. (0.7 oz.) tea, 454 gm. (1 lb) biscuits, 24 gm. (0.86 oz.) cocoa, 340 gm. (12 oz.) pemmican, 56.75 gm. (2 oz.) butter, and 85.12 gm. (3 oz.) sugar, a total of 980 gm. (2 lb. 3 oz.).

Amundsen's basic sledging ration per man and day was 400 gm. biscuits, 75 gm. dried milk, 125 gm. chocolate and 375 gm. pemmican, a total of 975 gm.

Scott's ration gave 4,430 Calories per man and day, Amundsen's 4,560 Calories. A healthy male doing manual work under normal conditions needs

Table 14.1

Scott's sledging ration for one man for one day

	kcals/oz	Barrier ration Wt.(oz)	kcals	Summit ration Wt.(oz)	kcals
Biscuits	108	14	1,512	16	1,728
Pemmican	167	8	1,336	12	2,004
Butter	226	2	452	2	452
Sugar lumps	112	4	448	3	336
Chocolate	160	1.43	229	—	—
Cocoa	128	0.86	110	0.57	73
Cereals	110	0.86	95	—	—
Raisins	70	0.86	60	A few on special days	
Tea: Leaves	17	0.57	0	0.7	—
Infusion	1	—	0	—	0
Totals		32.58	4,242	34.27	4,586

Barrier ration/day			Summit ration/day		
Protein	202g	828	Protein	257g	1054
Fat	178g	1,655	Fat	210g	1953
Carbohydrate	464g	1,740	Carbohydrate	417g	1564
kcal		4,223 approx.	kcal		4,571 approx

Vitamin Intake/day	Source	Barrier Ration	Requirements for work at 4,500 kcal/day	Summit Ration
Vitamin A and Carotene (i.u)	Butter	1,985	2,500 i.u. (i.e. 750 mg retinol equiv)	1,985
Vitamin D (i.u.)	Butter	22.7	100 (2.5 mg)	22.7
Tocopherois (mg)	Milk powder	4.7	Less than 20	5.2
Ascorbic acid (mg)	None	0	30 to 60	0
Thiamine (mg)	3/4 M.P.	0.93	1.8	0.88
Nicotinic acid(mg)	3/4 M.P.	8.09	29.7	8.28
Riboflavine (mg)	3/4 M.P.	1.26	2.4	1.24
Vitamin B12	M.P.	1	1 to 4	1.1
Folic acid (mg)	M.P.	25.6	100	29.3
Pyridoxine (B6) (mg)	M.P.	0.5	1 to 2	0.56
Biotin (mg)	M.P.	11.0	'a few mg'	12.6
Pantothenic acid (mg)	M.P.	3.5	3.5	4.0

M.P.: Skimmed milk powder in the biscuits. A quarter of the thiamine, nicotine acid and riboflavine came from the cocoa and chocolate allowance. Vitamin K, nicotine acid, riboflavine,
pyridoxine, biotin and probably pantothenic acid are synthesized in varying amounts by the
intestinal flora in man. The intense ultra-violet radiation would cause synthesis of vitamin D
in the exposed skin of the face. From: A. F. Rogers, "The Death of Chief Petty Officer
Evans," *The Practitioner* 212 (1974): 570–580.

about 3,600 Calories per day. On the return, Scott's ration decreased because of failing supplies, so that he was probably averaging under 4,000 Calories. From the 29th December, when Amundsen increased his pemmican allowance to 450 gm., he was getting 5,000 Calories. Scott probably needed about 5,500 Calories for the work he was doing, Amundsen, 4,500.

Scott's daily intake of thiamin was 1.26 mg., riboflavin, 1.65 mg., and nicotinic acid, 18.18 mg. The corresponding figures for Amundsen on his basic ration were 2.09 mg. thiamin, 2.87 mg. riboflavin and 25.85 mg. nicotinic acid, rising to 2.24 mg., 3.04 mg., and 29.3 mg. respectively, after the increase in pemmican. The accepted requirements for work at 4,500 Calories per day are 1.8 mg. thiamin, 2.4 mg. riboflavin and 29.7 mg. nicotinic acid. Lack of thiamin is associated with beri-beri; of nicotinic acid, with pellagra, both fatal if left untreated.[40]

Obviously, all values for the rations of these expeditions are estimates, because no analyses were, or could have been, made. Also, deteriorative chemical interactions could have greatly reduced the diet's nutritional values. For example, Rogers obtained data on the composition of Scott's biscuits that showed they contained sodium bicarbonate, which could have lowered the contents of some of the vitamins on baking, possibly destroying all of the thiamine.[41] Because the biscuits were an important source of thiamine, its possible loss could have been a critical deficiency, leading to incipient beriberi.

Some say that success breeds success, and that successful people are frequently crowned as victors. This really did not happen with Scott or with Amundsen. Amundsen got the credit for going to the pole first, but he was severely criticized for almost everything else he had done. As for Scott, his victory was in his death; Amundsen himself supposedly stated that Scott won by dying. But even Amundsen's countrymen were not at ease with his surreptitious change of objective from the north polar area to the South Pole. Naturally he became a national hero, but his glory was blunted by the lack of support from Nansen and a few other Norwegian notables. None of this occurred for Scott in England. He was not only a national hero but nearly deified as the personification of all that was great and glorious in British tradition—a British naval officer, a brave and intensive explorer, a seeker of scientific information while braving the worst conditions in the world, a man of irreproachable integrity. Most everyone would have to agree that this is all true.[42] Amundsen was a person whose only wish was to achieve the fame of getting to the pole first, and in order to do it he ate dogs. Englishmen would not do this any more than they would eat their fellow man, such as had been suggested during northern British explorations. As national heroes, Scott and his party were even a stimulus and a solace for the British military in World War I. Still, young men in Norway felt the strength of Amundsen and revered him in their own way.[43]

Both noted and hidden in the many versions and stories of these two expeditions are the nutritional reasons for their successes and failures.[44] Racing from depot to depot and killing his dogs, Amundsen not once appeared to be short of nutritious food. It is well known that Scott and his two companions were out of food when they died. Perhaps this has been overshadowed in history by the terrible storms and the time and energy taken for scientific observations and for the collection of specimens, but the difference was food. Also, underlying it all was what we now know, that food is metabolized and energy generated by the catalytic fires of vitamins and some trace metal ions. Aggravating this was the long time away from the home base where bodily storage of essential nutrients could have occurred from better food.

Notes

1. There have been many books, articles, and comments about these expeditions of both Scott and Amundsen. For Scott's primary sources, I have relied heavily upon *Scott's Last Expedition*, Vol. 1 and 2, arranged by Leonard Huxley (1913) and *The Worst Journey in the World* by A. Cherry-Garrard (1922), with help from *The Great White South: or with Scott in the Antarctic* by H. G. Ponting (1922) and *South with Scott*, by E. R. G. R. Evans (1921). For Amundsen's primary sources, I have relied upon *The South Pole*, Vol. 1 and 2 by R. R. Amundsen (1913), with help from *Voyages of a Modern Viking* by H. Hansson (1936).
2. L. Huxley, *Scott's Last Expedition*, Vol. 2 (London: John Murray Publishers, Ltd., 1913), 17.
3. L. Huxley, *Scott's Last Expedition*, Vol. 2, 63.
4. R. E. Priestley, "Inexpressible Island," *Nutrition Today* 4 (1969): 18–27.
5. L. Huxley, *Scott's Last Expedition*, Vol. 2 (London: John Murray Publishers, Ltd., 1913), 104.
6. Ibid.
7. Priestley, "Inexpressible Island," 24.
8. Ibid., 27.
9. Huxley, *Scott's Last Expedition*, Vol. 1, 120.
10. Priestley, 27.
11. Ibid.
12. Personal communication from Sir Charles Wright, 1964.
13. R. F. Scott, *The Voyage of the Discovery* (London: John Murray Publishers, Ltd., 1905), 709.
14. E. R. G. R. Evans, *South with Scott* (London: W. Collins Sons and Co., Ltd., 1921), 1.
15. L. Huxley, *Scott's Last Expedition*, Vol. 2 (London: John Murray Publishers, Ltd., 1913), 300.
16. Ibid., 406.

17. Ibid., 445.
18. R. E. Peary, *Secrets of Polar Travel* (New York: The Century Co., 1917), 44.
19. Huxley, *Scott's Last Expedition*, Vol. 1, 456.
20. B. J. Freedman, "Dr. Edward Wilson of the Antarctic. A biographical sketch, followed by an inquiry into the nature of his last illness," *Proc. Royal Soc. Med., Section of the History of Medicine* 47 (1954): 183–189.
21. Huxley, *Scott's Last Expedition*, Vol. 1, 463.
22. Ibid., 472.
23. R. E. Peary, "Brief Outline of a Project for Determining the Northern Limit of Greenland, Overland," *Civil Engineer USN*, National Archives (May 10, 1890): 4.
24. A. Cherry-Garrard, *The Worst Journey in the World* (London: Chatto and Windus Ltd., 1922), 554.
25. Ibid, 546.
26. R. Amundsen, *The South Pole* Vol. 1 (London: John Murray Publishers, Ltd., 1913), 44.
27. Since Peary had already discovered the North Pole and Amundsen was reputedly headed there again, there wasn't any value to Armour in supplying pemmican for the North Pole.
28. Amundsen, *The South Pole*, Vol. 1, 88.
29. Amundsen, *The South Pole*, Vol. 2, 59.
30. Ibid., 36.
31. Ibid., 159.
32. Ibid., 162.
33. Ibid., 178.
34. A. Cherry-Garrard, *The Worst Journey in the World*, 553.
35. A. F. Rogers, "The Death of Chief Petty Officer Evans," *The Practitioner* 212 (1974): 570–580.
36. Ibid., 578.
37. Evans, *South with Scott*, 207.
38. Rogers, 576.
39. H. E. Lewis, "State of knowledge about scurvy in 1911," in *Proc. Royal Soc. Med.: Section of the History of Medicine* 65 (1972): 39–42.
40. R. Huntford, *Scott and Amundsen* (London: Hodder and Stoughton, 1979), 545.
41. Rogers, 579.
42. During a sabbatical at the Scott Polar Research Institute at the University of Cambridge, England, I was impressed how its dignified and scholarly aura exemplifies the high regard that is today given to these British explorations. Visitors to London have missed an invaluable experience if they have not seen the *Discovery*. Boarding it, I could further sense the drive for achievement.
43. Visiting Tromso, Norway, I could feel the worshipful attitudes of the local people proudly surveying Amundsen's large statue in the square and pointing out the hotel where he stayed on his way to and from his voyages. On my visit to the *Fram* at Oslo, I could see that such a visit is a Norwegian youth's perfect holiday.
44. See Cherry-Garrard, *The Worst Journey in the World*; Amundsen, *The South Pole*, Vol. 1 and 2; Rogers, "The Death of Chief Petty Officer Evans"; and C. Neider, *Edge of the World, Ross Island, Antarctica* (New York: Doubleday and Co., 1974).

15

Douglas Mawson's Heroic Return

Douglas Mawson, born in Yorkshire, England, moved to Australia with his parents when he was two years old. His first experience in Antarctica was during Ernest Shackleton's attempt for the South Pole in 1908, where he served as a magnetician, cartographer, and surveyor. At this time he held a doctorate, he was a lecturer in geology at Adelaide University, and a big man of 6 feet 3 inches, a rough-and-tumble investigator of Australia's outback with extraordinary endurance. This he proved as part of Shackleton's three-man team that climbed the active volcano, Mt. Erebus, and as part of another team that went out seeking the south magnetic pole in an expedition to the northwest of McMurdo Sound.

After the Shackleton expedition, the antarctic bug had bitten Mawson so deeply that in January of 1910 he was in London meeting with Captain Robert Scott to consider going on Scott's next expedition.[1] Scott eventually invited him to be a member of the final team that would go for the pole. Mawson, however, rejected the invitation because there was a question as to whether he or Wilson would be the chief scientist on the expedition. With an intense interest in exploring Antarctica west from Cape Adare because of the proximity of this area to Australia and the possible great value of this exploration to his country, Mawson planned his own expedition. It left Hobart on December 2, 1911, in a very old Newfoundland sealer, the *Aurora*. After a difficult trip in which the ship was badly damaged en route, they made it into the antarctic southern ice pack by the end of December. Initially they could not get close to the antarctic shore and were actually driven somewhere about 800 miles west of Cape Adare. Continuing to sail west, they landed in what they later named Commonwealth Bay. Here Mawson set up his base, building what was to be the main headquarters for nearly the next two years.

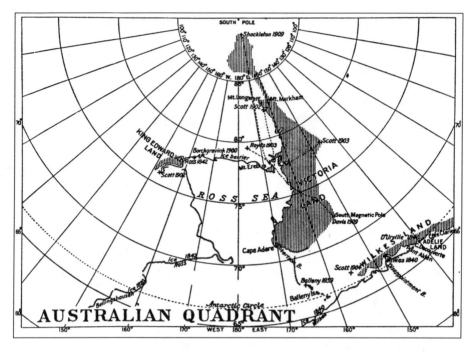

The Australian quadrant of the antarctic expedition before 1910. A. W. Greeley, 1910

After a very active antarctic winter making close-by runs, repairing equipment, and planning, they were ready and eager to leave in six separate teams:
(1) a Southern Party of three to do magnetic observations, (2) a Southern
Supporting Party of three for the Southern Party, (3) a Western Party of
three to traverse the coastal highlands, (4) a Near Eastern Party of three to
map the near eastern area, (5) an Eastern Coastal Party of three to map the
more easterly area, and finally (6) Mawson's party, the Far Eastern Party of
three, assisted by dogs. Mawson's party would travel not far from the coast,
yet would cover over 500 miles to plot the geography, claiming the land for
the crown. According to this plan, they would be able to go far enough
inland to see all the great sources of glaciers and possible treasures that
would be there for Australia. His two companions were Lt. Belgrave
Edward Sutton Ninnis of the British Royal Fusiliers and Dr. Zavier
Guillaume Mertz, a law graduate from Basel, Switzerland, a mountaineer
and skier. These three men were hardened and tough.

In outlining plans for the expedition, Mawson emphasized that food,
fuel, and shelter were the key elements. Their diet would be carefully

balanced for the heavy tough work ahead. Bags of rations were designed to give two pounds of dried food per day. He emphasized and greatly extolled the value of a hot "hoosh" from dried pemmican to cut the terrible hunger after a heavy work day. Added to it would be the niceties of chocolate, biscuits, sugar, cocoa, tea and sometimes dried milk. A few frivolities like raisins would be in their personal packs. For transportation Mawson's own party would have dogs, whereas the others would be man-hauling with some help from a converted smashed airplane: Mawson was the first to introduce an airplane into Antarctica, but unfortunately the wings were smashed by the ice, and then the men were only able to use it to jury-rig a device to help pull sleds part of the way for one of the other parties.

When the weather cleared, Mawson, Ninnis, and Mertz left on November 10, 1912. After stopping at a place they named Aladdin's Cave, which they had dug out of the ice as a stopping place for this and other expeditions, they were off. Mawson had calculated his supplies down to the last ounce. Food and fuel made up 1,260 pounds. Each of the men was to have thirty-two ounces of concentrated food per day. This was mainly pemmican and dried whole meal biscuits with some dried milk, sugar, cocoa, small amounts of cheese, chocolate and tea. Raisins were their extra food. Almost all of this was placed in a large water-proof bag giving a total weight of 500 pounds. Since the dogs needed to be fed as well, this added another 700 pounds of dried seal meat, blubber, and pemmican. Mawson had planned that the three men would have food for nine weeks, but what actually happened on this trip was far different, developing from one fatal disaster to another to a nearly final fatal disaster.

Almost all the food supply was on the last sledge, which was pulled by the best dogs. Mawson had reasoned that if they lost a sledge in a crevasse, it would be the first one, so that one should have the worst of the dogs and no food. It would seem that someone with Mawson's experience and knowledge would have divided his food more evenly between the sledges, but he put all his eggs in one basket: all the food and the strongest dogs with the last sledge. Mawson was a true dog man:

> There can be no question as to the value of dogs as a means of traction in the polar regions… Further, in an enterprise where human life is always at stake, it is only fair to put forward the consideration that the dogs represent a reserve of food in case of extreme emergency.[2]

On December 13 the party met with the first catastrophe. After seeing a faint indication of a crevasse, Mawson signaled to Ninnis, who was driving the rear sledge, and then went on. Then Ninnis was gone. Mawson saw nothing:

> When I next looked back, it was in response to the anxious gaze of Mertz who had turned round and halted in his tracks. Behind me nothing met the eye but my own sledge tracks running back in the direction. Where were Ninnis and his sledge?[3]

Ninnis, dogs, sledge, and food were gone into a deep crevasse. One-third of the party was gone, and most all of their food supply was lost. Only a bare one and a half weeks' worth of food was left for the two men, and nothing at all for the dogs. That night they made a thin soup by boiling up all the old food bags that could be found. The dogs were given some worn out fur mitts, finnesko, and several spare rawhide straps, all of which they devoured.

Only one option was left to them now, and that was to return. On the outward journey they had left no depots because they were going to make a circle on the way back, and they thought they had plenty of food. Not only were they essentially out of food, they had also lost most of their utensils and equipment. So they had to turn back.

On December 15 they reached one of their former camps, and here George, the weakest of the dogs, was killed and partly fed to the others and partly kept for the men. On the 17th they killed another and cut him up for supper. When the dogs were so miserable and exhausted, their meat was tough and stringy, without a vestige of fat. That night the men had only a few ounces of their stock of ordinary food, and to this they added a portion of the dog's meat. The major part was fed to the surviving dogs, who crunched the bones and ate the skin until nothing remained. On December 24 Mawson and Mertz wished each other happier Christmases in the future and divided two scraps of biscuit that Mawson had found in his spare kit bag, relics of better days. By the 26th they were eating mostly dogs' meat, to which was added one or two ounces of chocolate or raisins, three or four ounces of pemmican and biscuit mixed together in a beverage of very dilute cocoa. Two days later one of their favorite dogs, Ginger, could no longer walk and was killed and eaten:

> We had breakfast off Ginger's skull and brain. I can never forget the occasion. There is nothing available to divide it, the skull was boiled whole, then the right and left halves were drawn for by the old and well-established sledging practice of 'should I', after which we took in turns eating to the middle line, passing the skull from one to the other. The brain was afterwards scooped out with a wooden spoon.[4]

Now Mertz was definitely ill, his usual cheerfulness disappearing. He said that he felt the dog's meat was not doing him much good and suggested that they should give it up for a time. By January 1 Mertz did not complain at all except of the dampness in his sleeping bag, but when Mawson questioned him, Mertz did complain of abdominal pains. A few days later the skin was peeling off both of their bodies. Mawson remembered Mertz stating, "Just a moment," then reaching over and lifting from his ear a perfect skin cast. Mawson did the same for him, and there was hair and skin throughout their clothing. On January 7 Mawson had to help Mertz in and out of his sleeping bag. That afternoon Mertz died.

Alone, terribly sad, and dead tired, Mawson assessed where he was and his circumstances. Taking care of Mertz's remains and building the cairn had physically and mentally exhausted him, but he had to get going immediately. He wrote, "As there is now little chance of my reaching human aid alive, I greatly regret the inability to set down the coastline as surveyed for the 300 miles we travelled; and the notes on glaciers and ice formations, most of which is, of course, committed to my head."[5] Patching, sewing, and planning, he set about for the return, a return hastened by the terrible weather around him.

It was on January 11—a beautiful calm day of sunshine—that Mawson was able to start, but he was sore. Stopping to examine his feet he received a shock, for the thickened skin of the soles had separated, in each case as a complete layer, and an abundant watery fluid had escaped into his socks. Although there was new skin, it was already much abraded and raw. He was recognizing more and more his debilitated condition, but the sight of his feet was a blow to him because his feet were his only way to survive.

On the 17th, in overcast weather and falling snow, he was going on because delay meant a reduction in ration, which was already so very, very low. Then suddenly he was in a six-foot-wide crevasse, hanging freely in space, slowly turning around. Only after great effort was he able to bring a knot in the rope within his grasp and to draw himself up, reaching another. At length he hauled himself up on the overhanging snow ledge onto which the rope had caught. But he still had to climb carefully up the side onto the surface; then again he fell to the full length of the rope. Mawson almost gave up:

> It was a rare situation, a rare temptation—a chance to quit small things for great—to pass from the petty exploration of a planet to the contemplation of vaster worlds beyond. But there was all eternity for the last, and at its longest, the present would be short. I felt better for the thought.[6]

With his strength ebbing fast, he was able to pull himself out bit by bit and then lay for hours exhausted. Now he renewed his determination to make it out alive. Soon he set about making a ladder from alpine rope, one end of which was to be secured to the bow of the sledge and the other carried over his left shoulder and loosely attached to the sledge harness. Thus, if he fell again into a crevasse and the sledge was not engulfed, he would have a way of climbing out. Again and again he went into crevasses, but the sledge held back, and he said the ladder "proved trumps."

By the 19th he was off early, traveling across a network of crevasses, some very wide. The terrain turned better, but he wrote that he became over-confident and, in consequence, sank several times into narrow fissures. He knew the danger of despondency on the one side and over-confidence on the other. But pulling and pushing, with the sledge sometimes capsizing due to the strength of the wind, and finding it difficult to keep anything resembling an accurate course, he struggled on. On that day, when he pitched camp he reckoned that the distance covered in a straight line had been only about three and a half miles. On the 24th and 25th he was beset in a blizzard, and he wrote:

> I can not sleep, and keep thinking of all manner of things—how to improve the water, etc.—to while away the time. The end is, always food, how to save oil, and as an experiment I am going to make dog pem and put the cocoa in it. Freezing feet as too little food, new skin and no action; have to wear barberries in bag. The tent is closing in by weight of snow and is about coffin size now. It makes me shudder and think of the latter for the moment only.[7]

The tent was full of tufts of his beard and head hair. On the 26th he was off again, this time with a dense driving snow behind him so that he did not even use the sail he had. But the snow was in large rounded grains and beat down like hail. The good part was that he made nine miles. The next day the blizzard kept him tent bound again. Coming down from the 3,000 foot crest of a plateau, he found he was bearing down on Commonwealth Bay and began to feel that he knew where he was. Down to two pounds of food, he encountered a cairn of snow erected by a party who had come out searching for him. There was food there. On February 1 he reached Aladdin's Cave, safe but still far from surviving because he had to make it down to the hut. He was so close, and yet not out alive. A survey of his physical state gave a terrible picture. He had badly swollen joints full of fluid. His feet were terribly inflamed and oozing pus. All his nails, feet, and hands were

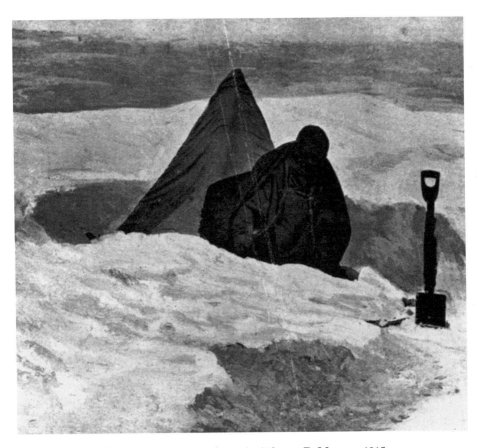

Mawson emerging from his makeshift tent. D. Mawson, 1915

broken about the swollen ends and filled with pus. Open cracks on his cheeks did not heal.

On his seventh day at Aladdin's Cave—the ice hole—he was still a captive of the weather as well as of his deplorable condition. Then the weather broke; weak and trembling, he slowly dressed and started off. Most everything about him had been made ready for this last attempt at survival. Several times he'd had to construct makeshift crampons, and he was wearing new ones made in the cave from boxes and nails. Going down the last trail he hauled his sledge, perhaps something he did not have to do, but he needed it desperately for the stability of his mind; it was a security blanket of the most personal kind. He thought the food at the cave had made him strong, so he was surprised at his weakness. A mile or so from the hut he looked down upon it and at Commonwealth Bay, and saw the ship leaving far off, an agonizing sight for him. This meant to him that he had missed it. Perhaps they had given him up for lost and he would have to spend nearly a year in this land alone. He wrote, "What does it matter? This terrible chapter of my life is coming to a close." But then he saw three men on one side of the boat harbor and he knew he was home.

Soon he was met by five men who had remained behind to search for his party. When they were all back at the hut, they made every possible effort to recall the *Aurora* by wireless. A forty-mile-an-hour wind was blowing across the bay right into the face of the *Aurora*, and there were dangerous ice cliffs to menace the ship. Even though the ship was still in the bay, the sea was so heavy that the motor-driven boat could never have lived through it. So they gave the ship's Captain Davis the option: He would have to decide either to stay on course or to return to the western base and pick up the party who would otherwise be left there for the winter, with much less equipment and facilities than were at the hut, perhaps condemning them to death. Later it was learned that Captain Davis never received the message but had acted on his own and sailed off. Mawson wrote, "The long Antarctic winter was fast approaching and we turned to meet it with resolution, knowing that if the *Aurora* failed us in early March the early summer of the same year would bring relief."[8]

Mawson's recovery was slow and painful during that long winter. Both then and many years later his friends saw that he never completely returned to his former state of health. A physician named McLean worked hard with him and could not understand what was wrong with him. When talking with newsmen the following year Mawson ventured a rare opinion about his condition:

> I know now the enforced isolation and in the hut for a second winter in that land was a blessing in disguise. My state was so poor, I was so near death's door, I now believe that had I been in time to board the *Aurora* and sailed immediately I could not have survived the long, rough sea voyage home.[9]

But yet he went on. In a note written by E. N. Webb entitled "An Appreciation" in Leonard Bickel's book, *This Accursed Land*, Webb wrote that when they met in New Zealand, Mawson had changed, but he still had some of his former self-reliance, strength, and purposefulness.[10] Changed he was, but it was for the better. Webb thought of him as superman, more humble and quieter. With perhaps the highest praise Webb could give, he believed the antarctic experience had made Mawson much closer to his God.

Mawson joined the service during the First World War and came back as a distinguished scholar in geology. In 1929–1931 he was back in Antarctica on Scott's old ship, the *Discovery*, when his expeditions established Australian interest in the antarctic over a vast sweep of the earth's surfaces.

What went wrong physically with the three on Mawson's trip? Ninnis' death was definitely a truly polar accident, but prior to that his physical condition had deteriorated. As the largest of them, he still ate only the same amount of food, he had a badly infected hand, and he had great difficulty in sleeping. With Mertz and Mawson there is very strong, if not almost irrefutable, evidence that their main illness was vitamin A hypervitaminosis, a toxicity from eating dog livers.

Many articles and notes have been written on the question of hypervitaminosis A in the Mawson expedition. Of these, three might be considered salient. The first, by Sir John Cleland and R. V. Southcott, was published in 1969.[11] Their summary stated, "It is considered that the illnesses of Mertz and Mawson in the far eastern sledging party of 1912–1913 are explicable as being due to hypervitaminosis A from eating husky liver after most of the other food supplies had been lost." In their discussion they said that in each case there was severe skin desquamation. In Mertz's case there were "fits" and other evidence of some major lesion of the central nervous system, as well as gastrointestinal manifestations. With Mawson there was hair loss and gastrointestinal symptoms such as abdominal pain. There did not appear to be any major evidence of extensive scurvy. Much later there was the demonstration of the high content of vitamin A in the livers of huskies and some seals from antarctic and subantarctic regions.[12] In the summary they stated, "Analyses of the vitamin A content of the livers of two species of seal and the introduced (domestic) husky in the antarctic or subantarctic regions are presented. The vitamin A content of the husky liver, *Canis familiaris*, indicates that the ingestion of about 100 grams of liver would be toxic to an adult."[13] Much of this was summarized still later by David J. C. Shearman in an article entitled "Vitamin A and Sir Douglas Mawson." Shearman analyzed the symptoms listed in Mawson's book, as well as his diaries:

> Mertz almost certainly died from hypervitaminosis A. The question of scurvy does not arise because no other member of the expedition suffered from it...Most of the six dog livers were probably eaten by Mertz and Mawson, and each liver would contain many toxic doses of vitamin A. The interesting question is why Mawson did not die also. He certainly suffered from hypervitaminosis A with desquamation with loss of hair and weakness.

> Possibly Mertz ate much more of the liver; he was a near vegetarian and the tough smelly dog meat might have been repulsive to him…Mawson's illness was characteristic of the chronic form of hypervitaminosis A rather than acute vitamin A poisoning.[14]

In comparisons with other clinically described cases of hypervitaminosis A, Shearman finds a close identity with Mawson's symptoms. He ends by saying, "His prolonged poor general health and slow recovery was in keeping with features in other recorded cases of chronic intoxication." What Shearman did not address was the effect of other problems from malnutrition that may have aggravated the vitamin A toxicity. So one of the last of the rigorous nonmechanized attempts to conquer the polar regions was devastated by poor nutrition.

Interwoven throughout the expeditions of Amundsen, Scott, and Mawson is the role that dogs played in their successes and tragedies. Amundsen most likely succeeded because he used dogs for transport as well as for food. Scott most likely failed because he did not use dogs. Some of Mawson's main problems have been attributed to eating dogs, including their livers. With Amundsen there was so much dog to eat that only the choicer cuts were consumed, while with Mawson there was so little dog to eat that he and his party ate every morsel or chewed every scrap of tendon. Whatever the outcome, dogs were the deciding factor.

Mawson, one of the last dog-sledging and man-hauling polar explorers, was also one of the first polar explorers to witness the explosion in the understanding of nutrition following the discovery of vitamins. At the time of his near-disastrous trip, he relied primarily on general medical advice, tempered with practical knowledge and common sense. There was nothing fancy about his writings on foods, just practical reality as he saw it:

> The subject of food is one which requires peculiar consideration and study. It is assumed that a polar expedition must carry all its food-stuffs in that variety and quantity which may approximately satisfy normal demands. Fortunately, the advance of science has been such that necessaries like vegetables, fruit, meats and milk are now preserved so that the chances of bacterial contamination are reduced to a minimum. A cold climate is an additional security towards the same end.
>
> Speaking generally, while living for months in an Antarctic hut, it is a splendid thing to have more than the mere necessaries of life…
>
> Luxuries, then, are good in moderation, and mainly for their psychological effect. After a spell of routine, a celebration is the natural sequel, and if there are delicacies which in civilization are more palatable than usual, why not take them to where they will receive a still fuller and heartier appreciation? There is a corresponding rise in the 'tide of life' and the ennui

of the same task, in the same place, in the same wind, is not so noticeable. So we did not forget our asparagus and jugged hare.

In the matter of sledging foods, one comes down to a solid basis of dietetics. But even dietetics as a science has to stand aside when actual experience speaks. Dietetics deals with proteins, carbohydrates, fats, and calories: all terms which need definition and comprehension before the value of a sledging ration can be fundamentally understood...

The proof of a wisely selected ration is to find at the end of a long sledge journey that the sole craving is for an increase in the ration. Of course, such would be the ideal result of a perfect ration, which does not exist.

Considering that an ordinary individual in civilization may only satisfy the choice demands of his appetite by selecting from the multifarious bill of fare of a modern restaurant, it will be evident that the same person, though already on the restricted diet of an explorer, cannot be suddenly subjected to a sledging ration for any considerable period without a certain exercise of discipline.

For example, the Eastern Coastal Party, sledging at fairly high temperatures over the sea-ice, noted that the full ration of hoosh produced at times a mild indigestion, they drank much liquid to satisfy an intense thirst and on returning to the Hut found their appetites inclined to tinned fruit and penguins' eggs. Bickerton's and Bage's parties, though working at a much higher altitude, had a similar experience. The former, for instance, could not at first drink the whole allowance of thick, rich cocoa without a slight nausea. The latter saved rations during the first two weeks of their journey, and only when they rose to greater heights and were in fine condition did they appreciate the ration to the full. Again, even when one becomes used to the ration, the sensation of full satisfaction does not last for more than an hour. The imagination reaches forward to the next meal, perhaps partly on account of the fact that marching is often monotonous and the scenery uninspiring. Still, even after a good evening hoosh, the subconscious self may assert itself in food-dreams. The reaction from even a short sledging trip, where food has been plentiful, is to eat a good deal, astonishing in amount to those who for the time being have lived at the Hut.[15]

In the appendix to his book Mawson made a detailed listing of the foods and their suppliers. Not only did he describe the foods but he also included reasons for their selections:

The food-stuffs were selected with at least as much consideration as was given to any of the other requisites. The successful work of an expedition depends on the health of the men who form its members, and good and suitable food reduces to a minimum the danger of scurvy; a scourge which has marred many polar enterprises. Thus our provisioning was arranged with care and as a result of my previous experience in the Antarctic with Sir Ernest Shackleton's Expedition.[16]

Probing east and west and along the coasts and toward the magnetic pole, Mawson extended the geographic coverage by his other teams as well

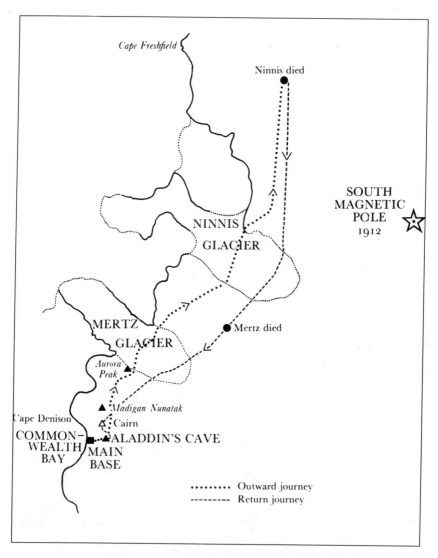

Mawson's path. Mawson's Institute for Antarctic Research,
Adelaide, South Australia

as by his own exploration. All of these made up a total picture, and fortunately the other teams did not meet with grim and tragic experiences like Mawson's.

The South Magnetic party, consisting of Bage, Webb, and Hurley, left Aladdin's Cave on November 10, saying good-bye to Mawson's party who were set to leave on their own sledging. Soon they met their supporting party and the six began pushing against a hard wind and thick drift, with winds of seventy to eighty miles per hour. On November 13, when the wind became mild—thirty-five miles per hour—they were off again. Breaking off from their support group, they continued against winds up to sixty miles per hour much of the time. Frequently making less than four miles a day, they struggled across sastrugi (wind-formed ridges of snow or ice, sometimes as high as several feet) of all types and thin crusts of ice which both feet and sledges broke through. Then on December 20 they realized that they had gone as far as they could. The farther land beckoned, although they knew it was the same featureless repetition and they were only 175 miles away from the spot where Mawson and his two companions had stood in 1909 on the Shackleton expedition. It was time to turn back. They were stopped by one thing—not enough food.

Being tent bound frequently, and just as frequently making only a few miles a day outward bound, they now had only enough rations for a return. With sixty-seven miles to go the food was proportioned to last for five days. "Dinner that night," according to party member Bage,

> consisted of a very watery hoosh, followed up by a mug of alcohol and water. We were all very thankful for the forethought of Dr. Mawson in providing absolute alcohol for lighting the primus, instead of methylated spirit. [Mawson himself used some on his trip.] Breakfast on the 9th was about the same consistency of dinner of the night before except that cocoa replaced the alcohol. In fact, breakfast was possibly even more watery as I was in charge of the food bag and surreptitiously decided to make the rations last six days instead of five.[17]

They just made it back to the hut on January 11.

The Eastern Coastal Party of A. L. McLean, P. E. Correll, and C. T. Mattigan headed out on November 8 together with their three-man support party. They holed up at Aladdin's Cave when they were weathered in by a good snow. What happened then has occurred over and over again in almost every part of the world: anoxia and perhaps some carbon monoxide poisoning from the lack of air. They frantically dug away the cave's entrance to save themselves—and they had not even really started on their journey.

On the 10th they started off, only for Correll to fall into a treacherous crevasse over sixty feet deep; luckily, suspended by his harness, he fell only six feet. After crossing paths with Mawson's group, they broke off with their support party and were on their way alone. Making a depot, they now took food for six weeks. With the going bad they had to attach themselves to an alpine rope in a long procession, a lucky decision because soon Mattigan was in a deep crevasse, hanging thirty feet down. His companions had anchored the rope to the sledge and so soon had him out to safety.

At a point 270 miles from the hut they made their farthest east camp on December 18, after a wonderful day's tramp of eighteen miles. Here, at a place they named Horn Bluff and Penguin Point, they started the first stage of their homeward journey.

Horn Bluff, rising out of the flat wilderness over which they had traveled, is a mammoth vertical barrier of rock, 1,000 feet high, and its whole face for five miles was like a magnificent series of organ pipes. Mattigan described it as "a cathedral of nature, where the still-small voice spoke amid an inevitable calm."[18] This beautiful area kept them working and entranced for several days as they moved along. Soon they were at what they named Penguin Point because there were a few penguins there, as well as hundreds of snow petrels and some skua gulls. On Penguin Point they found seals lying about, dozing peacefully, and Adelie penguins strutting in procession up and down the little glacier. Before leaving this mainland area they killed two penguins and cut off their breasts to use later for food. They made some good time until January 5 when again the weather hit. It was now fourteen miles to the top of a mountain they had to go over, and they had only two more days' rations and one and a half pounds of the penguin meat. Later, without any more food and with poor weather, they found that they didn't have the energy to haul the sledge up 1200 feet in three miles, which they had to do. But the weather cleared, and with the rest of the penguin meat, a half pound of it, the three ate a thin broth, the last they had. Mattigan, apparently the strongest, left the other two with the sledge and made the climb to the top to the depot. On his return McLean and Correll said they had felt the cold and were unable to sleep. In three days they had had only one mug of penguin broth. With food from the depot and some rest all was well, and they were off. By the 16th they were back at Aladdin's Cave, all safe and secured.

These other groups had none of the dreadful and fatal experiences of Mawson's own party. Nevertheless, again and again the controlling factor of their treks was the supply of food.

Notes

1. Most of the information and quotations in this chapter were taken from Douglas Mawson's very descriptive book, *The Home of the Blizzard*, Vol. 1 and 2 (London: Hodder and Stoughton England, 1914), and from the fine historical summaries and critiques of Mawson's diaries by the Jackas: F. Jacka and E. Jacka, eds., *Mawson's Antarctic Diaries* (London: Unwin and Hyman, 1988).
2. Mawson, The *Home of the Blizzard*, Vol. 1, 221.
3. Ibid., 239.
4. Ibid., 254.
5. Ibid., 260.
6. Ibid., 265.
7. F. Jacka and E. Jacka, *Mawson's Antarctic Diaries*, 165.
8. Mawson, *The Home of the Blizzard*, Vol. 1, 273.
9. L. Bickel, *This Accursed Land* (Melbourne: Sun Books, 1978), 198.
10. Ibid., 199.
11. J. Cleland and R. V. Southcott, "Hypervitaminosis A in the Antarctic in the Australasian Antarctic Expedition of 1911–1914: A possible explanation of the illnesses of Mertz and Mawson," *Medical Journal of Australia* 1 (1969): 1337–1342.
12. R. V. Southcott, N. J. Chesterfield, and D. J. Lugg, "Vitamin A content of the livers of huskies and some seals from Antarctic and subantarctic regions," *Medical Journal of Australia* 1 (1971): 311–313.
13. Ibid., 311.
14. D. J. Shearman, "Vitamin A and Sir Douglas Mawson," *British Medical Journal* 1 (1978): 283–285.
15. Mawson, *The Home of the Blizzard*, Vol. 1, 183–186.
16. Mawson, *The Home of the Blizzard*, Vol. 2, 314.
17. Mawson, *The Home of the Blizzard*, Vol. 1, 305.
18. Ibid., 335.

16

The Arctic and Antarctica After World War I

For some time after Mawson's explorations, much of the world was deeply involved in World War I, and most activities in the polar areas were restricted to minor naval forays. Soon after the war, however, men again were going south and north. Now the knowledge of vitamins struck down the previously held belief of many that scurvy resulted from spoiled food. Fresh foods could prevent scurvy as well as cure the disease. And it was believed that beriberi was also caused by a vitamin deficiency. These understandings affected the lives of polar explorers.

In 1917, Knud Rasmussen and two others explored the northwest of Greenland. Again there was starvation and exhaustion leading to the death of one of the three as well as an Eskimo helper. Later, Rasmussen, along with some Danish scientists, spent over three years (1921–1924) studying Greenland Eskimos. Many successful expeditions followed. Between 1926 and 1934 James Wordie completed several very successful arctic expeditions with few nutritional problems. Gino Watkins also led two successful arctic expeditions in 1930–1931 and again in 1932–1933, only to disappear when he went hunting in his kayak. Lack of food caused one arctic expedition to be disbanded in 1935 when a six-man expedition under Noel Humphreys became too dependent upon a group of Eskimos who were themselves short of food. In the south, most all went well.

Overland traveling was giving way to flying during the 1920s. From the aggressive seekings of William (Billy) Mitchell, the U.S. Army Air Force advocate for military air operations over the Arctic, came plans for polar flights.[1] Both sovereignty and national defense also strongly contributed to plans for U.S. arctic air bases. Of course, commercialization paralleled these motivations. Exploring and nature-studying were becoming less important.

With World War I over, both Amundsen and Mawson were again exploring. With Norway neutral during the war, Amundsen, like other Norwegians, made money in shipping, and so he had his own resources to continue probing into the Arctic. In 1918 he ventured to drift a ship, named the Maud, across the Arctic. This occupied several years though he did not achieve his main objective. Changing to air travel in 1925, Amundsen teamed with the American Lincoln Ellsworth and four others in an effort to fly from Spitsbergen to the pole. One of their two planes developed engine problems, and they spent nearly a month making an ice runway for an eventual escape. In 1926, at the age of fifty-four, Amundsen was the leader of the first transarctic dirigible flight. With financing from Ellsworth, he and his South Pole companion, Oscar Wisting, flew with the Italian pilot Umberto Nobile from Spitsbergen to Alaska. A successful flight occurred, in spite of a contention as to who would be in command: Nobile the airman or Amundsen the explorer. But they were not the first to reach the North Pole by air because Richard E. Byrd claimed to have been there several days before. Unfortunately for the claim, Bernt Balchen, the pilot on Byrd's flight over the South Pole, reported on his conversations with Floyd Bennett, Byrd's pilot over the North Pole. It was almost a death bed statement:

> He kept on licking his lips as he talked, and there was something he wanted to get off his chest, I could see that. Suddenly, he blurted out:
> It makes me sick to think of it.
> Think of what?
> That North Pole flight. If you knew the truth, it would shake you to your heels.[2]

If Byrd did not fly over the pole, then Amundsen would have had firsts at both poles.

In general, with regard to most attempts, success was considered just a minor enhancement. As long as there were no outright deceptions, the men involved were considered to have been engaged in heroic ventures; whether they missed the pole by a few miles was inconsequential.

Exploration by air, being short and quick, eliminated nutritional problems. The following year Amundsen published his book, *My Life as an Explorer*.[3] Far from being done as a leading polar explorer, and not to leave this world in an armchair, Amundsen was soon to make his very last venture. He attempted to rescue his former colleague and now competitor, Umberto Nobile, the captain of the airship *Norge*. Nobile had returned in another dirigible, the *Italia*, under the auspices of the Italian government in 1928. The *Italia* made it to the North Pole but did not land because of high winds and icing. On its return voyage to Spitsbergen it crashed. At least one person was killed on impact, and five others perhaps burned to death. When survivors, stranded on the ice, were able to transmit a radio message asking for help, several countries rushed to their aid.

A Swedish airplane rescued Nobile, but on returning for a second time the plane crashed and the crew had to join the isolated group on the ice. By this time three members, including a Swede named Malmgren, had taken off across the ice in order to seek help. Finally a Russian ship broke through the ice and found the survivors. The final toll was that twelve men died, including Malmgren in the three-man group. Of that group, only the two Italians returned; one was in great health and the other emaciated. Cannibalism was assumed by many, particularly by the Swedes, who were outraged that one of their citizens may have been eaten.

Amundsen was one of those who attempted a rescue. On June 18 he left Tromsø, Norway, in an airplane financed by the French government. Soon after take-off Amundsen and his two companions lost contact and were never found. They were counted as three of the twelve who died. Amundsen reputedly had said that Scott had won by dying. Perhaps Amundsen had, in the end, also won.

The rescue was tainted in three ways. One was that Nobile, the captain, was the first to be rescued. The second, germane to this subject, was evidence of some starvation and the possibility of cannibalism. The third was the loss of the hero Amundsen, a great loss to occur during a search for an expedition led by a competitor.

World War II brought extensive military activity and construction of military installations in Alaska, northern Canada, and Greenland. Some of these later became part of the United States' cold war defense early warning (DEW) bases. Food supplies at these bases were usually quite good because adequate transportation could bring in food which could be frozen and kept for long periods. As frequently may occur in far-flung military operations, there was some confusion in supplying the food but, in general, food was not only adequate but good. Cost was not a problem, of course.

As to the southern polar areas, between World War I and World War II many nations were active in and around Antarctica. Predominant among these were the United States, Norway, Germany, Britain, Australia, Argentina, and Chile. Mawson worked extensively in western Antarctica in

1929, and Admiral Richard E. Byrd had extensive activities from 1929 through the 1950s.

Byrd became America's latter-day counterpart of Amundsen and Scott. In 1929 he was in Antarctica and was the first to fly a plane over the South Pole. From 1933 to 1935 he established and occupied the U.S. base known as Little America. One trail ration designed by Dr. Dana Coman of the Johns Hopkins Medical School and a pemmican formulated by Professor Robert Harris show the then-current knowledge of nutrition (see table 16.1). During these times, Byrd contributed extensively to the modernization of antarctic travel, not only for airplanes, equipment and clothing but also for nutrition. As compared to today's knowledge, how little was known on these trail rations is seen in the report by Ernest E. Lockhard, a physiologist with the U.S. Antarctic Service:

> One of the newest fields in the science of nutrition is centered on the role played by vitamins. Vitamins have been known for some time and new accessory factors are still being discovered. The necessity of some vitamins in adult nutrition is now clearly understood. This is particularly true in the cases of vitamin C which prevents scurvy; vitamin A which aids, among other things, in keeping the repository tissue in health and in preventing night blindness; vitamin E, the reproductive vitamin; and some of the B vitamins which prevent nerve disorders and pellagra. The polar explorer is particularly interested in the availability of vitamin C in other than the normal sources, such as fresh fruits and vegetables, because he usually had to do without these. During recent years many vitamins in synthetic and concentrated forms have become popular at reasonable prices but these with the exception of vitamin C have had little opportunity for test in polar exploration.
>
> It was planned, therefore, that through the aid of synthetic and concentrated vitamin products, this special trail ration would provide adequate amounts of all critical vitamins. This is the first time in the history of polar explorations that the vitamin requirements of explorers were to be well taken care of.[4]

Certainly, the well-laid plans of Dr. Dana Coman guaranteed that adequate nutrition would be available for sledging operations, though the actions and decisions of the participants decided the outcomes. The writings of Dr. Lawrence M. Gould exemplify sound decision making. He led the ninety-day sledge journey undertaken by six members of Byrd's expedition.[5] This was the last antarctic expedition with dog teams and little possibility of a rescue in case of trouble. Gould believed that the most "prolific source of trouble and the commonest cause of failure, at least on the earlier sledging journeys, was improper food." In his book, *Cold, The*

Record of An Antarctic Sledge Journey he discusses his guiding factors in determining what supplies to include on this journey.

In devising a ration for a journey as extended as we expected ours to be, there were several guiding factors that we did not let ourselves forget or neglect. In the first place we had to get the greatest food value we could for the minimum weight (throughout all the details of our preparations even to such tiny items as a toothbrush, that old bugbear of weight could not be neglected) and with all have a balanced ration which would contain sufficient "roughage" and would be anti-scorbutic, that is would contain the necessary vitamin C which prevents that most dreaded of polar maladies, scurvy. Secondly, this ration should be composed of foods that would need little or no cooking. We had to carry all of our fuel, and fuel is heavy. Thirdly, so far as possible, some variation in the ration was highly desirable.[6]

With these notions in the background and largely due to the advice of Dr. Coman, the following ration [table 16.1] was worked out:

[Table 16.1]

Food Item	Daily Ration per man (ounces)	1 man for 90 days (pounds)	6 men for 90 days (pounds)
Pemmican	8	45	270
Biscuits	10	56.25	337.50
Sugar	4	22.50	135.0
Powdered milk	4	22.50	135.00
Oatmeal	2	11.25	67.50
Chocolate	2	11.25	67.50
Soup meal sausages	2	11.25	67.50
Tea	0.5	2.81	17.00
Bacon	1.33	7.50	45.00
Butter	0.59	3.33	20.00
Peanut butter	0.29	1.64	10.00
Malted milk	0.74	4.17	25.00
Cocoa	0.14	0.83	5.00
Salt	--	--	4.00
Pepper	--	--	1.00
Lemon powder	--	--	9.00
Matches and toilet paper	--	--	12.00
Totals	35.59	200.28	1228.00

The first group in the above [table] furnished the bulk or fuel part of our food, while the second furnished the desired variety. Furthermore the lemon powder was highly antiscorbutic.

Some of the above items [in table 16.1], perhaps, need a little explanatory comment. The pemmican was of Danish manufacture and the same kind that Amundsen had used with such success. It is composed essentially of finely ground dried beef and fats with a little seasoning. One pound is supposed to be the equivalent in food value of six or seven pounds of raw beef. The biscuits were in themselves a very good food, for they contained in addition to the natural wheat content, other vegetables and some meat. I found them more durable than edible—but strangely enough the former quality is a most essential one. If these biscuits were of the same consistency as ordinary soda crackers, they would get badly broken up and ground into powdery crumbs in the heavy handling they have to undergo. Considerable loss would be inevitable and it would be increasingly difficult to make an exactly equitable distribution or division into individual rations. The soup meal sausages were of the long famed German, "erbwurst" variety and made a most valuable and welcome addition to the pemmican.

Of all the food items [in table 16.1], the only one that really needs a good deal of cooking is oatmeal. One might at first thought assume that the amount of fuel necessary to cook the oatmeal would be so great that to take it along would be poor judgment. But we found that a large vacuum jug made an excellent fireless cooker and that it was only necessary to bring the oatmeal to a boil and then pour it into the jug after supper at night and leave it until morning. No matter whether it was 15 degrees above zero or 30 below, we always had steaming hot oatmeal for breakfast. Again the question arises as to whether the luxury of oatmeal for breakfast justifies the addition of so great a weight to our load as the vacuum jug. Had the jug served no other purpose we would not have let ourselves be persuaded to take it. But we worked out a scheme for travelling whereby it much more than made up for its weight, by the great amount of fuel it saved in other lines. We knew that we might be travelling anywhere from six to sixteen hours per day and that our loads would be so heavy that we could not at any time ride on the sledges. We realized that we had to plan to travel all the way on skis. Under such conditions it seemed very unwise to attempt a whole day of travelling without something to drink, at least. But the business of unlashing a loaded sledge and putting up a tent at noon time, so that we could have our stove lighted to melt snow for water, would have taken up a great deal of time, and would have greatly increased our fuel consumption. The vacuum jug saved us all this trouble. After breakfast, while the cooker was still hot, we brewed a jug of hot tea, cocoa, or malted milk. Thus we were able to stop for our noon day lunch and have two or three cups of some kind of hot drink, without causing much delay on the march.

We planned to distribute our ration through the three meals of the day as follows:

Breakfast: 2 mugs of oatmeal with sugar and milk
            2 biscuits
            2 cups of tea with sugar and milk

Lunch: 1 four ounce bar of chocolate
            2 biscuits with butter or peanut butter

> 2 ounces of pemmican (to eat cold)
> 2 cups of tea with lemon powder and sugar, or cocoa or malted
>   milk
>
> Supper: 6 ounces of pemmican made into hot stew or "hoosh" with
>   soup meal sausage
> 4 biscuits with butter, peanut butter, or bacon fat
> 2 cups of tea, cocoa, or malted milk
> 2 slices (thick) of bacon

Finally as a measure of convenience we packed our food supplies in bags, the pemmican and biscuits in bags, each containing rations for one day for the whole party, and the less bulky items like sugar in bags containing rations for one week. We made many of the heavy cloth bags, that I was taking for keeping my prospective rock samples separate, do double duty. We filled them with supplies that we expected to consume before we reached the mountains—that is, before they would be needed to hold rock specimens.[6]

Gould also had an improvisation of Nansen's cooker:

Since fuel was a fairly heavy item in our supplies, it is at once evidence that every means should be taken to see that it was used economically. The efficiency of the fuel is directly dependant upon the cooking arrangements. Though many devices have been tried, it has yet to be demonstrated that there is any more reliable and efficient type of burner for fuels in cold regions than the well-known primus stove. Our cooker was built around a two-burner primus stove and was constructed entirely in Little America by Victor Czegka. It was designed by him after the principle which Fridtjof Nansen had found so successful and efficient. We therefore called it the Nansen-Czegka Cooker.

It will be clear from the diagram just how the cooker operated. I don't believe a more efficient and a more handy arrangement has been devised for the kind of cooking that we had to do. Obviously the snow in the central pots melts long before that in the ring and top pots but only a small amount of water is formed from this original melting. Not enough to make our "hoosh." To avoid the task of taking the cooker apart to refill this pot with snow, and thus allow a considerable loss of heat, Czegka placed spigots in both the rig and top pots which made it an easy matter to draw the water off these pots and pour it down the funnel through the top pot into the central one. When the water in this pot began to boil the top pot was removed and the ingredients of our prospective hoosh were dumped in. It was ready to eat within three to five minutes. An extra pot identical with this central one was then filled with water and placed over the flames. The water in this pot became hot as we ate our stew and when it came to a boil we brewed our tea. Now as we drank our tea the emptied hoosh pot which had been filled with water was getting hot to cook the oatmeal. This water came to a boil about the time we were finishing our supper; the oatmeal was

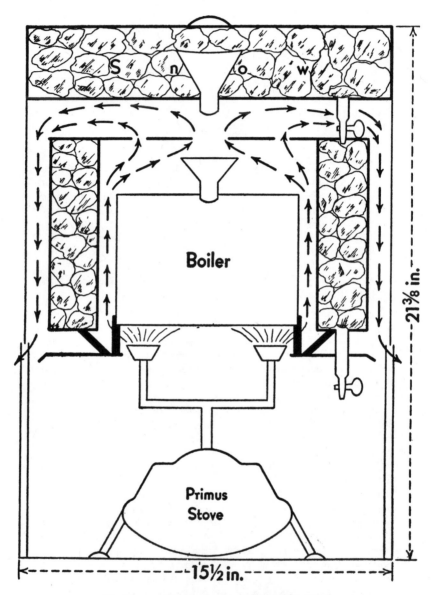

The Nansen-Czegka Cooker. L. M. Gould, 1931

dumped in and just allowed to come to a boil when it was poured into the vacuum jug.[7]

From 1939 to 1940, Byrd led a group devoted to scientific exploration. Byrd is best known to the general public for his flight over the pole in 1929 and for his lonely isolation in the Bolling Advance Weather Base, which he manned alone during the long antarctic winter nights of 1934.[8] For the first time in history there was extensive reliance on motor-driven tractors to haul material for an advanced base, but the tractors were found to need modifications and frequent repairs in the bitter cold. Though the original plan had called for a three-man team at the base, this had to be scrapped. Byrd finally had a choice of abandoning the plan or wintering by himself. He chose to be alone.

Byrd's five months of isolation is a modern epic. Certainly he did not have the long physical struggles of many of the earlier explorers, and he did have plenty of food, but he had other difficulties. Although he did not have a problem with toxicity from chemicals, he nearly died from carbon monoxide poisoning when problems occurred with his heating equipment.

His small quarters were prefabricated at Little America and tested by the now-well-experienced Paul Siple (the American Boy Scout selected from thousands to go with Byrd in 1929). He found out too late what was wrong with him: He became so ill that he could hardly move around, suffering from severe headaches and strange psychological feelings. Even though the condition was largely corrected, the prolonged toxic effects left him in a pathetic state. His communications with the main base indicated that something was radically wrong with him, and he agreed to be rescued. While waiting for the rescuing snowcat to reach him, Byrd took stock of where he was:

> This is the 61st day since the first collapse in the tunnel; nothing has really changed meanwhile; I am still alone. The men at Little America were no nearer, and all around me was the evidence of my ruin. Cans of half-eaten, frozen food were scattered on the deck. The parts to the dismantled generator were heaped up in a corner where I had scuffed them three weeks before. Books had tumbled out of the shelves, and I let them lie where they fell. And now the film of ice covered the floor, four walls and the ceiling. There was nothing left for it to conquer....[9]

But he made it and was rescued a few days later. Byrd was a naval officer, a good one, but prior to his arctic and antarctic work he was neither an explorer nor a mountain climber. He had a different nutritional shortcoming than many other explorers—he did not know how to cook.

His notes before the toxicity set in show his sense of humor and also his humility in admitting his lack of field experience being on his own; he had grown too accustomed to relying on others to do the cooking.[10]

Notes

1. N. Fogelson, *Arctic Exploration and International Relations 1906–1932* (Fairbanks: University of Alaska Press, 1992).
2. National Archives, Laurence Gould Collection, Correspondence, 1929–1971, RG 401(59), "The Strange Enigma of Admiral Byrd," by B. Balchen (1950).
3. R. Amundsen, *My Life as an Explorer* (Garden City, NY: Doubleday, Page and Co., 1927). In this autobiography we see Amundsen not just as an arctic and antarctic explorer, victorious so many times, but also as a man dealing with some sad feelings of loneliness and incompleteness. Perhaps this was due to haunting memories of the Amundsen-Scott race and Scott's death.
4. National Archives, Records of the U.S. Antarctic Service, Scientific and Technical Reports, Logs and Related Material, 1939–1943, RG 126, "Antarctic Trail Diet," Ms. No. 89, by E. E. Lockhert.
5. L. M. Gould. *Cold, The Record of An Antarctic Sledge Journey* (New York: Brewer, Warren and Putnam, 1931), 89.
6. Ibid., 74–78.
7. Ibid., 51.
8. R. E. Byrd, *Alone* (New York: G. M. Putnam's Sons, 1938). Just the title of his book, *Alone*, has sent many spines shivering. Located a little less than 150 miles from the main base at Little America, the weather base was still far enough away and deep in the Ross Ice Shelf area to supply much-needed information to go with that from the few other antarctic bases. This first recorded documentation of a voluntarily planned wintering-over vigil in the dark interior of Antarctica tugged at the imaginations of many and sometimes led to malicious gossip. There was even a rumor that the Washington, D.C., social whirl seriously considered Byrd to be a secret alcoholic who wanted to go off alone in a hole in the ice to drink. It was a long way from Washington to Antarctica, conceptually as well as physically.
9. Byrd, *Alone*, 204.
10. Ibid., 65.

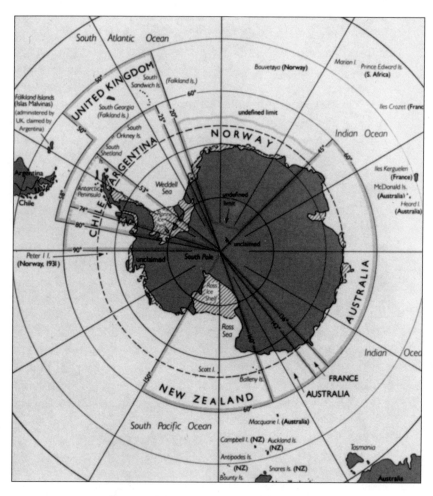

Territorial claims in Antarctica. S. J. Pyne, 1986

17

Antarctica Since World War II

During World War II the British were active in the South Orkney and South Shetland islands. Soon after the war, their activities in Antarctica accelerated rapidly. Three of the more famous expeditions were those led by Finn Ronne, Edmund Hillary, and Vivian Fuchs. Ronne, accompanied by twenty-one men and two women (one his wife), wintered-over in 1947–1948. In 1958 Hillary, using snow tractors, made the South Pole from Ross Island, and Fuchs made it all the way across Antarctica from the Weddell Sea to Ross Island. Great Britain and Argentina were so active in the Antarctic Peninsula that they became vigorously competitive, and still are. Both general interest in Antarctica and a concern about its protection caused many nations to discuss possible joint endeavors there. This resulted in the Third International Geophysical Year in 1957. The first had been in 1882–1883 and the second in 1932–1933.

The third was at both polar areas. Eventually seventy-six nations cooperated, with 12,000 scientists working at 2,500 stations. Polar work was no longer the strenuous life-threatening endeavor it had been. Air transportation was the main reason, followed by the wide use of treaded tractors, nicknamed snowcats. Heavy equipment and extensive supplies were still brought to coastal bases by ship during the proper season when possible.

The United States had already moved into the Ross Sea area and set up what became McMurdo base right next to Scott's first hut adjacent to the Ross Ice Shelf. The base was officially established in 1958. All of this could not have been done without the help of many of the earlier explorers, including Admiral Byrd, who was the honorary chairman, and Dr. Lawrence M. Gould, the geologist with Byrd in the early 1930s, who was chairman of

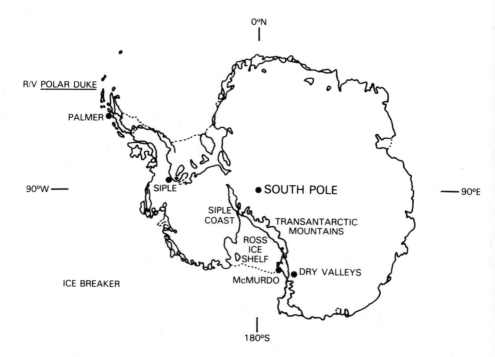

U.S. antarctic research programs, 1988–1989. National Science Foundation

the antarctic program of the U.S. for this International Geophysical Year. Finally, there was the south polar station itself, built and maintained by the United States and named the Amundsen-Scott Station.

During this time other nations also established stations, including the Japanese at Showa (on the west coast) and the Russians at Mirny on the Knox Coast, Vostok at the magnetic pole, and Sovetskaya at the Pole of Inaccessibility. While this was going on, the Antarctic Treaty of 1958–1959 was drawn up, an interesting treaty in that it was originally planned to bind its signatories for twenty-five years but has been extended.[1] The treaty was signed by Argentina, Australia, Belgium, Chile, France, Japan, New Zealand, Norway, the Union of South Africa, the Soviet Union, the United Kingdom, and the United States. It became effective in June of 1961. Since then many other nations have either added their names to the treaty or agreed to its covenants, and more may be added.

With the Antarctic Treaty in place at the beginning of the 1960s, extensive development in Antarctica began. Dedicated to peace and science, the Antarctic Treaty of 1961 promised that the spirit of the International Geophysical Year would continue.[2]

In 1964 McMurdo was a modern station in most all respects, though still beset with primitive conditions. A nuclear reactor was under construction for heating and distillation of sea water for drinking and other purposes. During the wintertime the base had around eighty personnel, whereas in the summer this could increase to more than 750. The base usually was opened for summer personnel around October 1, and it closed around March 1. Air transportation was the only type available until around Christmas, when icebreakers were used. The main buildings were of the World War II Quonset type, but there were several larger prefabricated metal buildings for equipment and other operational purposes. At that time personnel were housed entirely in Quonset huts except for one small prefabricated metal building which housed approximately a dozen people in small double sub-

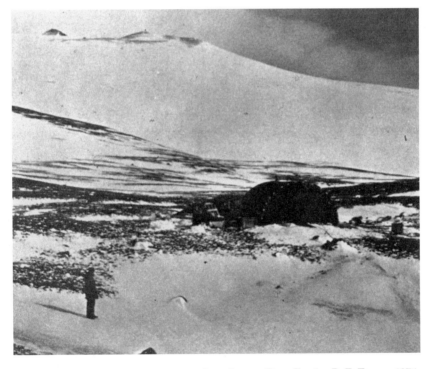

More modern living quarters near penguin rookery at Cape Crozier. R. E. Feeney, 1974

marine-type rooms. But even then there was no bath and no water. In fact, it was worse than being out in a tent because one had to hike over two blocks for water, any washing, and toilets. In a blizzard or with any illness, this was a long way. Getting around at McMurdo was also unpleasantly difficult, much more so than being out someplace else in a tent or Quonset hut. This was because of the large number of tractors and snowcats that used the roads, creating deep ruts with frozen earth or frozen ice that was often knife-edge sharp. Stepping and falling on these could cause serious injury. Although not a problem to the inhabitants, pollution was everywhere. Raw sewage was piped into the bay, and garbage and refuse were heaped on the ice for sinking when the ice melted.

Food there was in plenty. The personnel received four meals a day, including such choice items as lobster and prime steak.[3] Eating, however, was an operation rather than a pleasure at the main base. Facilities were in a very cramped Quonset hut, requiring that an individual eat quickly in order to make room for the next person. A large general utility building with a massive dining room and kitchen was constructed a few years later, which improved this situation.[4]

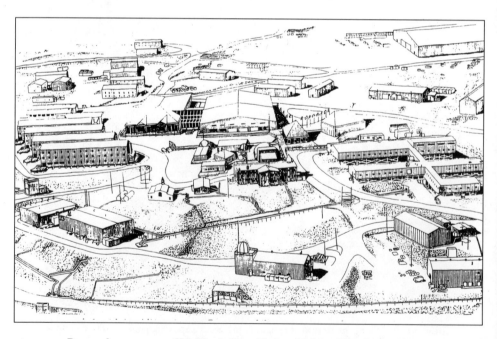

Proposed town center of McMurdo Base, National Science Foundation, 1994

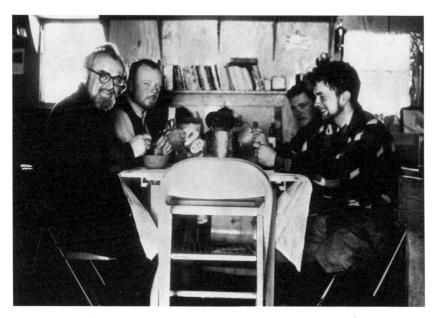

A more modern Thanksgiving dinner party in a hut at a penguin rookery, Cape Crozier, 1966. From left, author, Bob Wood, John Peterson, and John Boyd. R. E. Feeney, 1974

Field rations naturally varied considerably from those at the main base at McMurdo. Although frozen foods were usually no problem, canned and dehydrated items predominated. During the half-dozen years between 1964 and 1971 that my team worked at Cape Crozier, there was usually a team of three to five, and the job as cook rotated on a daily basis. Steaks, stews, and canned shrimp and lobster were prominent on the menu. Dehydrated vegetables were included, along with dried fruits, figs, prunes, raisins, apples, and apricots. Cereals, such as oatmeal, and puddings were everyday items. But the best of all was a daily diet of penguin eggs—cracked eggs only were gathered—discovered in the course of daily surveys of penguin colonies.[5]

In spite of the comparative comfort of modern living in Antarctica, there are still the grave dangers of the isolation and terrible weather. Probably the most serious danger is that of fire because there is no water away from the sea, and, to obtain even very small amounts of water, snow must be melted.[6] In some places, like Cape Crozier, the winds are well over 100 miles an hour and blow the snow off the volcanic rock, forcing long trips to get snow to melt for water.

With the great advances in food technology and knowledge of nutrition, the traditional food problems in Antarctica are now certainly minimal.

Differences that may occur are more likely to be man made than techno-logically caused. Even at McMurdo, there were many incidents when food was taken from the main supplies and eaten by small groups in private quarters. The diets of these men are not anything like what the nutritional surveys of the foods supplied would indicate. Certainly, although some such diets might even be excellent, the chances are that they were much worse nutritionally.

Facilities and the ways of life in Antarctica are continuing to be more like those at home. The McMurdo under development looks like a modern American town. As of 1994, university classes are held in January for students selected from many different universities. Reflecting the growing interest in Antarctica, the U.S. National Science Foundation, which oversees polar programs, elevated the status of the Division of Polar Programs by reclassifying it to the Office of Polar Programs, and placing it directly in the Office of the Director.

Notes

1. D. Shapley. *The Seventh Continent. Antarctica in a Resource Age* (Washington, D.C.: Resources for the Future, 1985).
2. R. E. Feeney, *Professor on the Ice* (Davis: Pacific Portals, 1974). My first-hand experience with Antarctica began in 1964, only three years after the beginning date of the treaty, when I worked at McMurdo and Cape Crozier on the other side of Ross Island, and then later at Cape Hallett.
3. This was because as much as ninety-five percent of the cost of the food was due to transportation, so it made little difference whether it was lobster or second-grade hamburger.
4. The food improved as well and was twice as healthful. See table 17.1 (page 200–201) for a typical menu. The quantities were unlimited. The midnight meals were more truncated on the published list, but often they might contain foods left from the evening dinner, and so could be as sumptuous as the other meals. Likewise, eating at some of the larger summer-operated outstations improved materially, even with full-time professional cooks. Although small isolated encampments might cook up stews as before, their supplies could contain some of the currently available supermarket delicacies.

   Between 1964 and 1971 I was in Antarctica six different times, doing research at McMurdo, Cape Crozier, and Cape Hallett. Usually the team included four to five coworkers, most of whom were graduate students. During my first three visits, there were no women. Now a welcome change is the presence of women, who make up an appreciable percentage of the cadre at the main base.

   The work was split between the main base, tent huts, and fishing houses far out on the ice. Changing and growing, McMurdo was like an Alaskan gold rush camp, although run by the U.S. military and the National Science Foundation, with many scientists struggling to get started on their research. About 100 yards up the hill was the installation called "Nukiepoo," the nuclear power plant to generate heat, but mainly used for melting snow and attempting to distill sea water for the everyday serious need to provide fresh water. It was both here and at some of the planning conferences that I met many of the antarctic old timers with whom in a few cases, I became close friends.

5. We daily found up to half a dozen cracked eggs. These we could take for food. A little fishy, yes, but otherwise excellent for omelets and fine for fried or boiled eggs when one became accustomed to the difference in their properties as compared to chicken eggs. Penguin eggs are like some other water birds' eggs in that the egg white becomes translucent on cooking, rather than opaque like chicken egg white and the yolk cooks to more of a jelly-like consistency. For more information, see R. E. Feeney et al., "Biochemistry of the Adelie Penguin: Studies on Egg and Blood Serum Proteins." *Antarctic Res. Series* 12 (1968). Reprinted from *Antarctic Bird Studies*, J. R. Austin, ed., O. L., American Geophysical Union.

6. Just using an ordinary Coleman camp stove for cooking was found to be a danger. Once the whole thing caught fire and we were just able to get it outside in time to prevent the tent from going up in flames. This was during a storm, which would have made it very difficult for any rescue operations. In another incident, a large barricade built of 4 x 8s and heavy planking was erected behind the tent hut because of the very strong winds that howled down from Mt. Terror. In one such wind this huge barricade broke off and blew over the tent, just missing us by a few inches. Still, both life and food were good, and there was even a Thanksgiving banquet one year.

Table 17.1
Weekly menu for the U. S. Naval Support Force Antarctica, McMurdo Station, Antarctica—Cycle One

Breakfast

MONDAY	TUESDAY	WEDNESDAY	THURSDAY	FRIDAY	SATURDAY	SUNDAY
Assorted Cold Cereal	Assorted Cold Cereal	Assorted Cold Cereal	Assorted Cold Cereal	Assorted Cold Cereal	Assorted Cold Cereal	Assorted Cold Cereal
Hot Buttered Farina	Hot Buttered Oatmeal	Hot Hominy Grits	Hot Buttered Farina	Hot Oatmeal Cereal	Hot Hominy Grits	Hot Buttered Farina
Fried Eggs to Order	Fried Eggs to Order	Fried Eggs to Order	Fried Eggs to Order	Fried Eggs to Order	Fried Eggs to Order	Fried Eggs to Order
Fried Omelettes to Order	Fried Omelettes to Order	Fried Omelettes to Order	Fried Omelettes to Order	Fried Omelettes to Order	Fried Omelettes to Order	Fried Omelettes to Order
Grilled Sausage Slices	Grilled Sausage Links	Grilled Ham Slices	Grilled Canadian Bacon	Minced Beef on Toast	Hot Corned Beef Hash	Grilled Sausage Patties
Grilled Ham Slices	Grilled Bologna Pinwheels	Grilled Bacon Slices	Grilled Sausage Patties	Grilled Ham Slices	Grilled Sausage Links	Grilled Ham Slices
Grilled Bacon Slices	Grilled Bacon Slices	Cream Dried Beef	Grilled Bacon Slices	Grilled Bacon Slices	Grilled Bacon Slices	Grilled Bacon Slices
Hash Brown Potatoes	Hash Brown Potatoes	Hash Brown Potatoes	Hash Brown Potatoes	Hash Brown Potatoes	Hash Brown Potatoes	Hash Brown Potatoes
French Toast with Syrup	Strawberry Pancakes	French Toast with Syrup	Hot Griddle Cakes	French Toast Puffs	Blueberry Pancakes	Thick-Slice French Toast
Cheese Biscuits with Cream Gravy	Breakfast Pastries	Breakfast Pastries	Breakfast Pastries	Breakfast Pastries	Breakfast Pastries	Scotch Woodcock
Breakfast Pastries	Asst. Jams, Jellies	Asst. Jams, Jellies	Asst. Jams, Jellies	Asst. Jams, Jellies	Asst. Jams, Jellies	Breakfast Pastries
Asst. Jams, Jellies	Hot Maple Syrup	Coffee, Tea, Milk	Hot Maple Syrup	Hot Maple Syrup	Hot Maple Syrup	Hot Maple Syrup
Coffee, Tea, Milk	Coffee, Tea, Milk	Coffee, Tea, Milk	Coffee, Tea, Milk	Coffee, Tea, Milk	Coffee, Tea, Milk	

Lunch (Sunday Brunch)

MONDAY	TUESDAY	WEDNESDAY	THURSDAY	FRIDAY	SATURDAY	SUNDAY
Chicken Noodle Soup	Vegetable Supreme Soup	New Engl. Clam Chowder	Cream of Mushroom Soup	Oriental Egg Drop Soup	Tomato Vegetable Soup	Onion & Mushroom Quiche
Grilled Ham Steaks	Spicy Barbeque Spareribs	Baked Fillet of Fish with Tartar Sauce	Savory Chicken Adobo	Beef Sukiyaki	Hot Turkey Gravy	Hot Sloppy Joes
Baked Tuna with Noodles	Braised Pork Spareribs	Grilled Salisbury Steaks	Breaded Veal Steaks	Tempura Fried Fish with Tartar Sauce	Braised Pork Chops with Savory Bread Dressing	Crispy French Fries
Candied Sweet Potatoes	Simmered Knockwurst with German Sauerkraut	Golden Macaroni & Cheese	Steamed Egg Noodles	Oriental Fried Rice	Hot Whipped Potatoes	Baked Pork and Beans
Simmered White Beans with Ham Hocks	Shrimp Fried Rice	Hot Franconia Potatoes	Steamed Green Rice	Oven Baked Potatoes	Seasoned Green Peas	Salad Bar Assortment
Seasoned Mixed Vegetables	Cottage Fried Potatoes	Seasoned Peas & Mushrooms	Seasoned Asparagus Spears	Fried Fresh Cabbage	Corn O'Brien	Dessert Bar #7
Southern Style Cornbread	Steamed Garden Peas	Baked Yellow Squash	Carrots Normandie	Seasoned Wax Beans	Hot Dinner Rolls	Asst. Cold Beverages
Salad Bar Assortment	Fresh Brown & Serve Rolls	Hot Dinner Rolls	Hot Cream Gravy	Hot Fresh Dinner Rolls	Salad Bar Assortment	Coffee, Tea, Milk
Dessert Bar #1	Salad Bar Assortment	Salad Bar Assortment	Fresh Hot Dinner Rolls	Salad Bar Assortment	Dessert Bar #6	
Asst. Cold Beverages	Dessert Bar #2	Dessert Bar #3	Salad Bar Assortment	Dessert Bar #5	Asst. Cold Beverages	
Coffee, Tea, Milk	Asst. Cold Beverages	Coffee, Tea, Milk	Dessert Bar #4	Asst. Cold Beverages	Coffee, Tea, Milk	
	Coffee, Tea, Milk		Asst. Cold Beverages	Coffee, Tea, Milk		
			Coffee, Tea, Milk			

Table 17.1 (continued)
U.S. Naval Support Force Antarctica, McMurdo Station, Antarctica—Cycle One

	MONDAY	TUESDAY	WEDNESDAY	THURSDAY	FRIDAY	SATURDAY	SUNDAY
Dinner ("Sunday Dinner Delight")	Hot Navy Bean Soup	Hot French Onion Soup	"Amore Italiano": Steaming Minestrone Soup	Hot Beef Barley Soup	Split Pea Soup with Ham	Turkey Rice Soup	Hot French Onion Soup
	Yankee Pot Roast with Hot Natural Gravy	Baked Seasoned Meat Loaf	Simmered Italian Pasta with Beef Spaghetti Sauce	Roast Loin of Pork with Hot Pork Gravy	Savory Roast of Lamb	Golden Roast Duckling	Grilled Steak to order
	Savory Baked Chicken	Braised Liver with Onions	Baked Hot Italian Sausage	Stuffed Frankfurters	French Fried Shrimp with Cocktail Sauce	Hot Ham & Noodle Casserole	Sauteed Onions & Mushrooms
	Parsley Boiled Potatoes	Hot Mashed Potatoes	Assorted Pizza Pies	Fresh Lyonnaise Potatoes	Hot Mashed Potatoes	Oven-Glo Potato Slices	Fried Rice with Vegetables
	Steaming White Rice	Seasoned Oriental Rice	Assorted Cold Cut Platter	Vegetable Fried Rice	Baked Rice L'Orange	Simmered Brussel Sprouts	Steamed Corn on the Cob
	Herbed Green Beans	Seasoned Spinach Leaves	Cauliflower Au Gratin	Scalloped Creamed Corn	Seasoned Carrot Pennies	Cauliflower Polonaise	Seasoned Green Beans
	Glazed Garden Carrots	Seasoned Corn Niblets	Hot Garlic Bread	Seasoned Green Beans	Baked Club Spinach	Hot Baked Cornbread	Salad Bar Assortment
	Hot Fresh Baked Rolls	Hot Brown Gravy	Salad Bar Assortment	Finger Rolls	Hot Vegetable Gravy	Salad Bar Assortment	Dessert Bar #7
	Salad Bar Assortment	Hot Baked Dinner Rolls	Dessert Bar #3	Salad Bar Assortment	Hot Dinner Rolls	Dessert Bar #6	Asst. Cold Beverages
	Dessert Bar #1	Salad Bar Assortment	Coffee, Tea, Milk	Dessert Bar #4	Salad Bar Assortment	Asst. Cold Beverages	Coffee, Tea, Milk
	Coffee, Tea, Milk	Dessert Bar #2	Coffee, Tea, Milk	Asst. Cold Beverages	Dessert Bar #5	Coffee, Tea, Milk	
	Asst. Cold Beverages	Asst. Cold Beverages		Coffee, Tea, Milk	Coffee, Tea, Milk		
		Coffee, Tea, Milk					

From U.S. National Science Foundation

18

Space Exploration

Space offers new frontiers, even in the realms of diet and nutrition. In only thirty years space scientists have made many trips, some lasting for only weeks, although one lasted as long as a year. Current plans are for colonies living in space for as long as two years and for people to travel in exploring probes.

Proper nutrition is as important to those engaged in space exploration as it was to polar explorers.[1] Space travel is dependent on modern technology, including computers and guidance systems, but without proper nutrition, modern technology will not ensure a successful manned mission. Further, proper nutrition cannot be achieved without knowledge of the foods that will provide the nutrition. Scientists thus are challenged to achieve further advances in providing suitable foods. Ultimately, findings from research in food technology will be used to establish a self-contained environment in space, where waste products will be recycled and crops and even some forms of animal food may be raised.

The United States' space program has completed several phases of space travel. First space capsules were launched, up for a few hours or even days. Then there were space shuttles, the Russians' space station, and the U.S. planned space stations. In the future, perhaps true biospheres will exist in space. The ideas and technology for such oases in the sky originate in the United States primarily from the National Aeronautics and Space Administration (NASA), private companies, and universities. Likewise, in Europe and Japan similar studies are underway. By 1996, 350 persons have been in space world wide. One, Story Musgrave at age sixty-one, has completed his fifth time in orbit. And then there is Ms. Shanon Lucid, a scientist and a mother, who in 1996 completed 188 days in space.

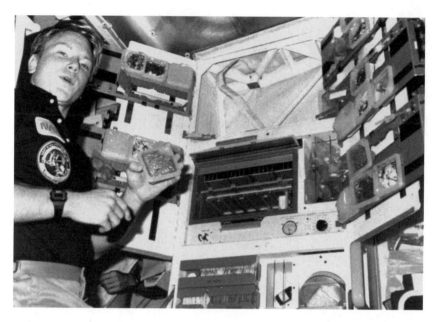

Astronaut George Nelson in space station galley. NASA

Since the beginning of the space program experiments have been conducted to determine if life can be maintained for long periods in a contained environment. First, there were the Mercury and Gemini flights. Then, in the late 1960s, came the Apollo program and the U.S. landing on the moon. These were followed by the joint United States-Soviet Union flight in 1975, the Apollo-Soyuz test project (ASTP). In 1981 the launch of the U.S. space shuttle Columbia marked the beginning of an era in the history of manned space flight. Columbia was launched as a rocket, orbited Earth as a space craft, and landed as a glider. Now on multiple flights, including operational missions with scientists aboard, there are up to a total of eight astronauts.

Early U.S. astronauts did not eat too well. John Glenn found eating was easy, though unpalatable. In early Mercury flights, food was consumed as bite-sized cubes, freeze-dried powders, and semiliquids in aluminum tubes. Water was sipped through a straw from a plastic bag. The freeze-dried foods were hard to rehydrate and caused another problem—crumbs, which floated in the air and fouled up instruments, which had potentially dangerous consequences. By the Gemini missions, squeeze tubes were gone, the bite-sized cubes were coated with gelatin to reduce crumbling, and the freeze-dried foods were placed in special plastic containers for easier reconstitution with water.[2] The menu even included items such as shrimp cocktail, chicken, vegetables, and butterscotch pudding. By the time of the Apollo flights, improvements continued to be made. Hot water made rehydrating the dried foods easier and tastier. Skylab brought yet further improvements, including a special dining area, food warmer, refrigerator, and freezer.

By the time of the shuttles some of the simpler hurdles had been overcome, but the remaining problems were monumental. The first was the tremendous amount of weight and volume that the foods occupied when supplies were needed for longer periods. Microbial contamination had to be prevented and the foods had to be easy to prepare and consume. And, of course, the foods had to be attractive and certainly nutritious. When weight and volume are considered, an important factor is water. In the space shuttle

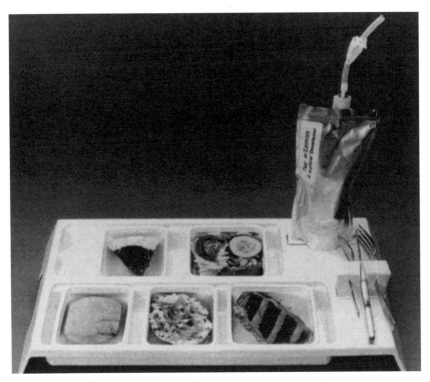

Dinner on a meal tray for space station food system. NASA

this was not a problem because electricity was supplied by combining hydrogen and oxygen in fuel cells, and the by-product was water.

As with everything else in micro or zero gravity, special procedures were required for the preparation and eating of foods. The limited supply of electricity prevented the use of microwave cooking because of the need for large surges in power. When a liquid is left in an open container it can float away and, due to surface tension, become a floating ball. So special procedures had to be developed for drinking fluids and for rehydrating dehydrated foods.

On the space shuttle food is prepared in a galley installed on the mid deck. For a typical meal, food is held inside separate containers on a meal tray. Crew members can attach a tray to their laps with a strap or can attach it to a wall. It is both the dinner plate and an exhibit from which to choose what to eat first. The individual foods are in plastic-covered containers inserted into places on the tray; the astronaut opens the top of the plastic and eats the food directly. The only thing unusual is that the plastic must be cut open to get at the food. Knives, forks and spoons are attached to the tray magnetically. Little time is needed for preparation of the food; a full meal for a crew of four can be set up in about five minutes. Dehydrated food requires extra time to reconstitute. Food for a four-day cycle is listed in table 18.1.

Over half of the total food items in earlier space shuttles were dehydrated food and powdered beverage products. Since there was no difficulty with a source of water, these were preferable. A variety of powdered beverages were supplied. As can be seen in table 18.2, nonbeverage dehydrated foods made up nearly a quarter of the total foods in the earlier flights. They included soups, casseroles (chicken and rice), shrimp cocktail, breakfast items (scrambled eggs and breakfast cereals), and freeze-dried bananas and pears. During earlier flights, the dehydrated foods were packaged in transparent plastic pouches called "Apollo Spoonball" packages. The rehydration of these was a problem, though, and they were replaced by square nestable package shapes that fit directly into the eating trays. Other foods included cookies and granola bars, heat-processed items either wrapped in aluminum or in cans, some intermediate-moisture foods taken down to low enough moisture that microbial action did not occur, and some meat and bread products sterilized by irradiation. A few fresh foods were added and could be used for the first few days. All in all, the astronauts enjoyed an adequate diet.

Living in space for three months or longer involves a gamut of special problems not found on briefer trips. First, everything must be on board for

Table 18.1
Standard 4-day menu cycle for the U.S. space shuttle

Meal	Day 1[a], 5	Day 2, 6	Day 3, 7	Day 4, 8
A	Peaches, Diced	Applesauce	Peaches, Dried	Apricots, Dried
	Beef Patty	Dried Beef	Sausage	Granola w/Blueberries
	Scrambled Eggs	Granola	Scrambled Eggs	Breakfast Roll
	Bran Flakes	Breakfast Roll	Cornflakes	Vanilla Inst Breakfast
	Cocoa	Chocolate Inst Breakfast	Cocoa	Grapefruit Drink
	Orange Drink	Orange-Grapefruit Drink	Orange-Pineapple Drink	
B	Frankfurters	Corned Beef	Ham	Grd Beef w/ Pickle Sauce
	Turkey Tetrazzini	Asparagus	Cheddar Cheese Spread	Noodles & Chicken
	Rye Bread (2x)	Rye Bread (2x)	Rye Bread (2x)	Stewed Tomatoes
	Bananas	Pears, Diced	Green Beans & Broccoli	Pears
	Almond Crunch Bar	Peanuts, Dry Roasted	Crushed Pineapple	Almonds
	Apple Drink (2x)	Lemonade (2x)	Shortbread Cookies	Strawberry Drink
			Cashews	
			Tea w/Lemon & Sugar (2x)	
C	Shrimp Cocktail	Beef w/BBQ Sauce	Mushroom Soup	Tuna
	Beef Steak	Cauliflower w/Cheese	Smoked Turkey	Macaroni & Cheese
	Rice Pilaf	Grn Beans w/Mushrooms	Italian Vegetables	Peas w/Butter Sauce
	Broccoli w/Cheese	Lemon Pudding	Vanilla Pudding	Peach Ambrosia
	Fruit Cocktail	Pecan Cookies	Strawberries	Chocolate Pudding
	Butterscotch Pudding	Cocoa	Tropical Punch	Lemonade
	Grape Drink			

a. Day 1 (launch day) consists of Meals B and C only.

Table 18.2
Types of food used in the U.S. space shuttle food system

Food Type	Total Items Sent	Food System Composition %
Irradiated Food	609	3
Fresh Food	1,333	6
Intermediate Moisture food	1,894	8
Thermostabilized Food	3,385	14
Natural Form Food	3,532	15
Rehydratable Food	5,289	22
Rehydratable Beverages	7,677	33
Total	23,719	100

the whole period or the space station must be resupplied at intervals. So far they have been resupplied. Next, social interaction must be considered, since the crews who are contained in close quarters for long periods must get along with their fellow travelers. The psychological aspects of life in space have been given serious consideration.[3]

The Russians have made a prolonged flight of 364 days in space. In his book, *Diary of a Cosmonaut: 211 Days in Space*, Valentin Lebedev vividly describes the many aspects of his long space flight. Lebedev, whose title was flight engineer V, was aboard with only one other astronaut. He stated that a daily diet consisted of about two-thirds freeze-dried foods and was varied on a six-day cycle of four meals a day. They were allowed 1.7 liters of water each per day. Electric heaters were used to warm the food inside cans, tubes, or plastic bags. On the station a snackbar-type system was installed and stored behind panels on both sides of the station. There were freeze-dried soups and natural liquid soups such as borscht and solianka (soup like a hash) in tubes. Their favorite foods were cottage cheese, beef, pork with potatoes, various meat dishes, poultry, canned fish, coffee, tea, milk, and various natural or sublimated juices. They had eight different types of bread. Crumbs were apparently a problem, and some of the breads had to be con-sumed in bite-sized cubes. He stated that they could eat whenever they so desired and sometimes just chewed on goodies. (See tables 18.3 and 18.4.) Foods were maintained by frequent resupplies, which also gave them a chance to be with other people for short periods.[4]

The United States program for its space station Freedom is still in the planning stage. NASA's Johnson Space Center in Houston, Texas, has created a model of the portion of the station that will be occupied by workers.[5]

Valentin Lebedev's descriptions of his 211 days in space might make it seem that feeding astronauts in space for long periods would be a simple task. This might be the case, depending on the individual and the condi-tions. As a general practice and certainly as a basis for longer periods, however, extensive planning is essential. Charles T. Bourland, a NASA scientist, and his colleagues stated that the goal is to provide choices that are both appealing and nutritious. Three different food systems are planned: (1) the daily menu food supply, (2) special foods for in-suit use during space walks, and (3) extra foods called "safe haven" in case of emergencies.[6]

For the daily food supply, NASA plans to provide a diet like that available on Earth. The arrangement is for a fourteen-day food supply that

Table 18.3
List of the food items on the Salyut-7 station

Baked Products
1. "Stolovy" bread (whole wheat bread)
2. "Borodinskiy" bread (bread with anise)
3. Moscow rye bread
4. White wheat bread
5. Honey gingerbread

Canned Food
6. Rib steak
7. Perch savoury
8. Beef tongue
9. Perch à la Polish (a fish in white sauce)
10. Ham
11. Chopped pork ham with egg
12. Bacon
13. "Liubitelskaya" sausage (bologna)
14. Cold cuts
15. Liver paté
16. Chicken with prunes
17. Cheese Rossiyskiy
18. Creamed goose liver
19. Karbonat (similar to beef jerky)
20. Quail paté
21. Quail with egg
22. "Azu" (meat with vegetables)
23. Beef with mayonnaise
24. Veal with vegetables
25. Jellied sturgeon
26. Sturgeon in jellied tomato sauce

Food in Aluminum Tubes
27. Green "stchi" (soup with sorrel)
28. Borscht with smoked meat

Food in Aluminum Tubes (continued)
29. "Stchi" with sauerkraut
30. Cottage cheese with black currant puree
31. Cottage cheese with apple
32. Cottage cheese with cranberry
33. Vegetable tomato sauce, "Moldova"
34. Black currant juice with sugar
35. Apple juice with sugar
36. Cherry-apple juice with sugar
37. Cranberry-apple sauce
38. Vegetable "caviar"
39. Cherry juice with sugar
40. Cranberry beverage

Freeze-Dried Food Items
41. Thick vegetable soup
42. Soup: "khartcho" (very spicy soup with rice)
43. Borscht with meat
44. Broiled beef with mashed potato
45. Pork sirloin with mashed potato
46. Golubtsy (cabbage leaves stuffed with meat)
47. Beef à la Tallin with mashed potato (pot roasted beef)
48. Home cooked beef (pot roasted beef)
49. Stew with vegetables
50. Cottage cheese with nuts
51. Cottage cheese with wild strawberries
52. Pasteurized milk

Freeze-Dried Food Items (continued)
53. Buckwheat hot cereal
54. Mashed potato
55. Sauteed cabbage
56. Black currant nectar
57. Cherry juice nectar
59. Apple nectar
60. Apricot juice nectar
61. Apple-black currant nectar
62. Acidophilus paste with high fat content
63. Sweet yogurt
64. Peach-black currant nectar and glucose
65. Strawberries
66. Aerovit multivitamins

Pastries
67. "Kunjut" candies
68. Hard melting chocolate "Osoby"
69. Sugar cookies "Sakharnyoe"
70. "Arktika" biscuits
71. "Russkoye" cookies
72. Dried apricots
73. "Vostok" cookies

Other Food Items
74. Prunes with nuts
75. Apple and plum fruit sticks
76. Prunes
77. Quince fruit sticks
78. Fruit dessert, plums and cherries
79. Tea with sugar
80. Coffee with sugar
81. Tea without sugar
82. Apple and apricot fruit sticks
83. Fruit dessert "Stelutsa"

From: Lebedev, V. 1988. *Diary of a Cosmonaut: 211 Days in Space*, Phytoresource Research, Inc. (in cooperation with the Gloss Co.), College Station, Texas (translated from Russian).

Table 18.4
Daily menu of a cosmonaut on board Salyut-7

	Food Item	Wt(g)	Net Water	Protein	Fats	Content (g) Carbo	Energy Value
Breakfast	1. Bacon	100	61.8	17.6	13.6	4.7	211
	2. Mashed potato	50	2.5	4.0	9.2	30.1	212
	3. Borodinsky bread	45	18.9	2.9	1.0	21.0	99
	4. Fruit dessert, plums & cherries	50	12.5	1.6	—	32.6	128
	5. Coffee with sugar	24	—	—	—	20.0	75
	Sub Total	269	95.7	26.1	23.8	108.4	725
Lunch	1. Savoury perch	100	70.0	18.0	7.0	1.3	140
	2. Hard biscuits "Arktika"	25	2.4	2.4	2.6	17.6	98
	3. Peach & black currant nectar	45	1.3	—	—	37.8	142
	Sub Total	170	63.7	20.4	9.6	56.5	380
Dinner	1. Quail paté	100	59.8	17.3	20.4	0.04	254
	2. Meat borsch	30	1.5	6.0	4.5	14.0	117
	3. Beef à la Tallin with mashed potato	52.5	2.6	18.4	7.9	16.7	207
	4. Moscow rye bread	45	18.9	2.9	1.1	20.7	99
	5. Quince fruit stick (50)	12.5	0.5	—	34.2	130	—
	6. Pasteurized milk	25	1.0	6.4	6.3	9.9	119
	Sub Total	302.5	96.3	51.5	40.2	95.9	926
Evening Snack	1. Asst. cold cuts	100	60.8	17.8	10.6	8.8	200
	2. Cottage cheese with currants	165	85.1	13.5	22.6	40.6	410
	3. Wheat bread	30	9.6	2.7	2.3	15.0	87
	4. Tea with sugar	46	—	—	—	—	150
	Sub Total	341	155.5	34.0	35.5	104.4	847
Snack	1. Vegetable "caviar"	82.5	52.0	3.3	11.1	11.5	157
	TOTAL	1165	473.2	135.3	120.2	276.7	3035

Tomato Sauce "Moldova" and Apple Cranberry Sauce. One "Aerovit" vitamin pill should be taken twice daily.

From: Lebedev, V. 1988. *Diary of a Cosmonaut: 211 Days in Space*, Phytoresource Research, Inc. (in cooperation with the Gloss Co.), College Station, Texas (translated from Russian).

could be changed from the logistics module, which in turn would be replaced every ninety days. But even with this fourteen-day schedule there is a built-in procedure to make a daily change in the planned menu, in case an individual at the last minute, just before food preparation, wants something different. The psychological aspect of food is an important consideration. Not only is food important psychologically; if food were rejected it would pose problems in trash management.

As in Antarctica today, the original cost of items pales when considering the dollar value of delivery. Of the many things that have to be considered, Bourland and coworkers particularly have focused on half a dozen, among which are: (1) Ease of preparation. Time spent by the crew in preparing food will detract from their other activities and thus will be very expensive time, so a high priority must be given to ease of preparation and clean-up. (2) Water. The water on board will be limited. Some recycling of water on board the Freedom is planned, but in contrast to the shuttle system where water is formed as a by-product from the vehicle's electricity-generating fuel cells, the water used for food rehydration and drinking will have to come from Earth. This reduces the amount of dehydrated food that can be used. Frozen and thermostabilized (canned, etc.) foods will make up an appreciable amount of the supply. (3) Food packaging. A modular packaging system is recommended in which the width of all packages is held constant so they will fit in the storage containers, the galley oven, and the meal trays. Some items, such as bakery products, however, will be packaged in bulk. (4) Food system logistics. For a ninety-day tour of duty by eight astronauts 2,160 meals would be stowed on board. Assuming that an average meal (including snacks and beverages) contains an excess of six containers, there would therefore have to be about 14,000 food packages. All of these must be stored and distributed in racks. (5) In-flight food preparation and service. Much of NASA's proposed approach for this is drawn from what was done on the shuttles. Trays with utensils attached to magnets are to be fastened either to the individual or to appropriate places. Each of the items in the tray would be covered by plastic prior to serving.

In addition to all of this, some fresh food will be carried aloft under refrigeration and would be useful for at least up to a week. Also there is a plan to develop some hydroponic cultivation to supply fresh vegetables, an aspect of food provision limited by the constraints of time and space, which must be balanced against the crew's psychological well-being.

Of all the goals for space living, the one that is most imaginative, and perhaps is nearly the ultimate goal, is what has been called the biosphere.[7]

The biosphere would contain a bioregenerative life support system that would supply almost all of its crew members' needs, with the exception of concentrated vitamins. Energy would come from the sun and waste products would be reutilized. A biosphere would be very different from a space station like Freedom. Because of the long periods its crew would be away from Earth, there would need to be more comforts and more people. Some of the refinements intended for a space station would probably not be available in the developmental stages of the biosphere. Only in science fiction has anything like it been achieved so far.

It is not known when a successful space station can be established, but certainly it is decades away. Extensive research and planning have been conducted for some time and are actively pursued.[8] General problems that will need to be overcome include the ever-prevailing existence of micro or zero gravity that affects most everything. The gravitational environment of a space station, and possibly of a trip to Mars, is at the microgravity level, while gravitational forces on the moon are about one-sixth that on Earth, and Mars' surface gravity is about one-third of Earth. At this time there are no simple ways for alleviating the gravity problem. One possibility would be to put the human occupation part of the biosphere at the ends of long arms swinging from a hub—an induced gravitational force caused by centrifugation. This clearly presents many engineering and other challenges. Without alleviating the gravitational problems, other information must be gathered as to how plants and humans exist for long periods in low gravitational forces.

As with polar explorations, the food supplied will determine the success or failure of the mission. Water will be a critical need, of course, as will oxygen. Some of this can be provided by recycling. But recycling will not entail simply purification. In the case of foods it means the use of organic waste products for supplying the needs of the plants and animals to be used as food. Solar energy, waste carbon dioxide, recycled water, and mineral elements will provide for the growth of photosynthetic organisms that in turn will provide food, oxygen, and transpired water. Thus the complete biosphere system must be capable of continuously recycling almost every-thing needed by the processing of waste and the regeneration of essentials.

All of this will not be accomplished until researchers have found the answers to many questions. First there are the effects of low- or microgravitational conditions. How would different kinds of plants grow under low gravity? Even on Earth little is known on the processing of waste to be used to grow foods. Bioreactors for bacteria and algae must be studied.

Should plants be grown in solid material, such as artificial soils, or should they be grown in hydroponic conditions? On Earth some bacteria can harm plants. How would these be controlled in space? Plant scientists will be a very important part of the biosphere's successful development. Then there is the need to maintain a healthful environment. The air must be uncontaminated, with the transpired carbon dioxide kept at a proper level and all the gaseous human waste products removed. Even volatile substances coming from foods and personal toiletry have already been found to accumulate and must be properly controlled.

If food is to be produced in-house, certain foods must be omitted from the diet because of the difficulty in producing them in a biosphere. Beef and pelagic marine fish such as tuna or swordfish are obvious examples. On the other hand, poultry and eggs are candidates for inclusion, but most of the foods will necessarily be of plant origin. This will require special processing to ensure a variable and acceptable diet.

Food and nutrition, and the technology of making food appealing as well as nutritious, will be a cornerstone of the biosphere. In selecting foods both the requirements for the majority of the party and for particular individuals will have to be considered. Even with careful screening of candidates for the spacefaring crew, some differences may appear. Low bulk should be advantageous in reducing volumes of human waste, but this could affect elimination. Very little is known about how well people will fare in such close quarters and isolated from the outside world. Engineering and physical science will provide the mechanism, but food will sustain the individuals who live in it.

Biosphere 2 is the name given to an experiment currently in progress in Arizona.[9] Biosphere 2 is described as: "a 3.15 acre space containing an ecosystem that is energetically open (sunlight, electric power, and heat) but with air, water and organic material recycled." With a nearly vegetarian diet the eight biospherians were initially slated to be healthier physically after a year inside than before they started. All these nutritional studies, however, were judged eventually to be improperly done, and the human experimentations were stopped in 1994.

> The cultish fantasy shattered completely in April 1994, when the enterprise's backer, Texas oil heir Edward P. Bass, called in marshals to eject the former managers who had inspired the project and put his $200 million structure in the hands of scientists. Now under the control of a consortium that is led by Columbia University's Lamont-Doherty Earth Observatory, Biosphere 2 is fitfully searching for a scientific identity.[10]

Now under new management, Biosphere 2 is to be used for hard-core science primarily related to the study of a controlled ecosystem.[11]

Even when living in space is achieved, on other planets as well as in orbit, there would be many problems in the handling and processing of foods. NASA has been studying these in detail:

> The Controlled Ecological Life-Support System (CELSS) program organized by NASA aims to develop safe life-support systems in space, consisting of biomass production, food processing, waste treatment, atmosphere regeneration and water purification. Space-effected change in weight and volume management, plant performance and microbial behavior affect food processing in space. Scientists should understand the role played by gravity and influence of space on heat and mass transfer. CELSS should integrate all the subsystems and develop more efficient processing and waste treatment methods.[12]

Will the spirits of the great polar explorers be with the space explorers of the future? Future astronauts may have to spend decades or even lifetimes away from Earth. Will they be expert scientists as well as having the fervors of Scott, Amundsen, Shackleton, Mawson, Nansen, Peary, Franklin, both the Rosses, Perry, and others? Will they be able to improvise as needed? To be creative? Or will they have to be automatons following exact directions? If so, they could develop boredom, which could affect their lifestyles including their selections of foods and consequently their nutrition. Will the space explorers conquer the intricate physical operations only to die from starvation?

Notes

1. H. W. Lane, "Nutrition in Space: Evidence from the U.S. and the U.S.S.R.," *Nutrition Reviews* 50 (1992): 3–6.
2. "NASA Facts," NF 150/1-86 (U.S. National Aeronautics and Space Administration, 1986).
3. See A. A. Harrison, Y. A. Clearwater, and C. P. McKay, *From Antarctica to Outer Space* (New York: Springer-Verlag, 1990). See also the symposium proceedings, "The Human Experience in Antarctica: Application to Life in Space," sponsored by NASA and the Division of Polar Programs of the National Science Foundation, Washington, D.C. The opening sentence of the proceedings states: "The overall goal of the proposed conference is to promote renewed efforts to conduct innovative, high quality behavioral research pertaining to psychological and social adaptation to Antarctica and, by analogy, to outer space and other isolated and potentially harsh environments."
4. V. Lebedev, *Diary of a Cosmonaut: 211 Days in Space* (College Station, Texas: Phytoresource Research, Inc. in cooperation with the Gloss Co., 1988).

5. As one of many visitors given the hospitality of a tour by the center, I could easily see the work that had gone into the planning. A diagram of the operational centers showed their compactness and interrelated parts. Designed for a crew of eight, the members will live in what is called a habitation module where the general living and eating facilities will be located. There will be individual laboratory modules for the U.S., the European Space Agency, and the Japanese National Space Development Agency. Consumable food items will be replaced with each crew change at ninety-day intervals.

6. C. T. Bourland et al., "Designing a food system for Space Station Freedom," *Food Technology* 43, 2 (1989): 76–81.

7. See J. W. Tremor and R. D. MacElroy, "Report of the First Planning Workshop for CELSS Flight Experimentation," *NASA Conference Publication 10020*, (Washington, D.C.: U.S. National Aeronautics and Space Administration, 1988.)

8. Ibid.

9. See R. L. Walford, S. B. Harris, and M. W. Guniun, "The Calorically restricted low-fat nutrient-dense diet in Biosphere 2 significantly lowers blood glucose, total leucocyte count, cholesterol, and blood pressure in humans," *Proc. Natl. Acad. Sci USA* 89 (1992): 11533–11537; R. G. Hahn, "Expedition to Another World: Biosphere 2 Crew Completes Mission One," *Explorers Journal* 71 (1993): 161–167; and R. L. Walford, "A Scientist Reflects on His '21st Century Odyssey' within Biosphere 2," *The Scientist* (January 21, 1994).

10. T. Bearsdley, "Down to Earth, Biosphere 2 Tries to Get Real," *Scientific American* 273, 2 (1995): 24–26.

11. G. Tauber, "Biosphere 2 Gets New Lease On Life From Research Plan," *Science* 267 (13 January 1995): 169.

12. B. Fu and P. E. Nelson, "Conditions and constraints of food processing in space," *Food Technology* 48 (1994): 113.

conclusion

Food and Exploration Today

For thousands of years, explorers either had to keep their trips short or make frequent stops to replenish supplies. Some nutritional help was obtained by carrying live animals aboard, but these were cumbersome, troublesome, and subject to dying untimely. In surveying the long history of exploration, a reader finds few substantial advances on foods and nutrition—with just two exceptions—until the first part of the 20th century.

The two exceptions were James Lind's findings in the value of lemons for treatment of scurvy and Nicholas Appert's development of canning. Dr. Lind's reports in the 1750s on lemon juice for treating scurvy could have had an early and far-reaching effect, but unfortunately, his recommendations were usually followed incorrectly or not at all. Then there was the interpretation that acidic solutions (e.g., carbonated water) were adequate substitutes for lemon juice. The cause of scurvy, a vitamin deficiency of ascorbic acid, was not recognized by the time of the early 1900s explorations of Robert Scott and his contemporaries. Scott even believed that scurvy was caused by spoiled foods.

Common sense, traditions, and cultural practices together were, therefore, the main basis for some good foods and nutrition for explorers before the beginning of the 20th century. After Scott's time, and by the end of World War I, came the early beginnings of the appreciation of the roles played by vitamins. By the time of Byrd in the early 1930s, some vitamins were identified. Between 1930 and 1940 there was an explosion in the knowledge of vitamins. This led to nearly adequate diets for the U.S. military and is the basis for today's understanding of the relationship between food and proper nutrition. Certainly, little evidence of poor foods and nutrition accompanied the extensive developments in Antarctica following World War II.

Running through the many problems of earlier explorations is a continuous line of difficulties caused by people, in particular those at the higher level of administration, but field leaders caused their share as well. Sometimes, inferior foods were purchased at lowest bids or by avaricious purchasing officers at ports of call. Then there were the large naval ships carrying as many as 400 men; provisioning these ships by stopping at islands was impossible, for there simply was not enough fresh food available for so many men.

Equipment for handling and preparing food also did not change much until the 20th century, with the important exception of the development of canning in the mid-18th century. Canning seems an unremarkable process today, but at the time, this was a great advance. Ships became better able to push through the ice when adequately equipped with motor-driven propellers (first with side wheels). But not until the advent of wireless telegraphy (and later radio) and then the airplane could explorers hope to be rescued if accidents occurred or they were out of food. And much of this technology was not fully developed until well into the 20th century. Now, except for sportsmen, dogs are not usually used, having been replaced with motorized snow tractors and snowmobiles.

Almost all of the advances in food and nutrition, transportation, and safety did not come from the needs of polar explorers. The needs of the military and just ordinary people were the main forces that drove the developments. Canning, one of the primary developments, exemplifies this: it was developed to win a prize for supplying food for French naval vessels. Canned, evaporated milk was another such development.

Newer military rations, such as the Meal Ready to Eat (MRE), have been adapted for civilian (i.e., sportsmen) use.[1] These rations contain a cooking element that heats the components when water is added. Unfortunately, their acceptance in the Gulf War was poor. General H. Norman Schwartzkopf, commander-in-chief of the allied forces, described the MRE as "an unappetizing glob of thermoprocessed food in a plastic pouch...they looked and tasted like paste..."[2] As with the K ration of World War II, the MRE suffered from overexposure during the Gulf War. Although standards dictated that the MRE could only be fed as a sole source of food for periods of ten days or less unless supplemented, the U.S. units relied upon them for months on end with little other food to break the monotony.

Research and development continues for improving food and nutrition in space.[3] Foods for space missions are researched and developed at the Food Systems Engineering Facility at the NASA Johnson Space Center.

Food scientists, dieticians, and engineers work together. Foods are examined through nutritional analyses, sensory (taste, physical feeling, etc.) evaluation, tests for how well they hold up in freeze drying and rehydration, observation of storage effects and packaging suitability, and many other methods.

Space is the next frontier, and the next main advances in food and nutrition may well be for space exploration. Self-contained environments (biospheres) would be necessary for people living for long periods in space. In addition to the many requirements for food production and all the other critical conditions for human habitations, the food that is grown will have to be processed for consumption—that is, food technology will have to come into play, for food technology in space is very different from that on earth.[4] The big problem is reduced, and even zero, gravity in space ships. As gravity is reduced, phenomena such as buoyancy, settling, convections, mixing, and diffusion are considerably changed. These affect heat transfer and bubble behavior, just a few of the actions altered: space explorers may make surprising discoveries without ever leaving their kitchens. Earth-based food technological processes are designed to take advantage of gravity effects. Perhaps microgravity could be used to advantage, but the problems are so many that "there is a long way to go before food processing will actually occur in space."[5]

Notes

1. R. E. Feeney, E. L. Askew, and D. A. Jezior, "The Development and Evolution of U.S. Army Rations," *Nutrition Reviews* 53, 8 (1995): 221–225.
2. R. Moore, personal communication for observations while on service as an officer in nutrition research. U.S. Army at Desert Storm, 1991. See R. E. Feeney et al., "The Development and Evolution of U.S. Army Rations."
3. NASA Facts, *Food for Space Flight*, National Aeronautics and Space Administration, Lyndon B. Johnson Space Center, NP-1996-07-007JSC, July 1996. See also B. Fu and P. E. Nelson, "Conditions and Constraints of Food Processing in Space," *Food Technology* 48, 9 (1994): 113–127.
4. Fu and Nelson, 113–127.
5. Ibid., 126.

appendix a
Descriptions of Nutrition

In the early part of this century, two scientists did the research that led to the name "vitamin," then called "vitamine." Gowland Hopkins worked with rats and purified diets and showed that the addition of very small amounts of different foods to some diets had a greatly beneficial effect on the growth and health of the rats. At about the same time, Casimir Funk coined the term "vitamine," and put forward the idea that the diseases scurvy, pellagra, rickets, and beriberi were vitamine deficiencies. Soon it was shown that there were a number of different vitamines, and eventually the "e" was dropped from vitamine when it was known that they were not related to the chemical substances amines. A turning point occurred in 1915 when E. V. McCollum showed that both fat-soluble (termed "A") and water-soluble (termed "B") substances were essential. This was just the beginning of a long trail of discovery of many vitamins. Along the pathway were many scientific high hurdles that had to be surmounted and many seemingly anomalous findings even when the finish line had been reached. A scientific puzzle, later so easy to understand, was that the vitamin A in fats was found by some workers to be yellow-colored and by others to be colorless. An argument developed. Eventually it was shown that the colorless vitamin A of some workers was the vitamin A, or retinene as we now know it, found in cod liver oil and some other animal products. The yellow-colored materials with vitamin A activity were present in plants and are now known as carotenes. In the animal body the carotenes serve as precursors of vitamin A. At this time vitamin A was the one known fat-soluble vitamin, whereas vitamin B included all the water-soluble ones. Soon vitamin C was reserved for the antiscorbutic agent, now known as ascorbic acid. Then there occurred the splitting of the fat-soluble vitamins into two types, vitamins A and D. Vitamin A was shown to be important for vision and for some skin characteristics, while vitamin D was important for the utilization of calcium in bone growth. Early experiments were necessarily done under restricted conditions because vitamin D is synthesized in the skin by action of the sun on cholesterol derivatives present in the skin. In other words, man and other animals can synthesize their own vitamin D under optimal conditions.

Still later, in the 1930s, niacin, or nicotinic acid as it is sometimes called, was found to be the vitamin necessary to prevent pellagra. Again difficulties arose along two separate but related lines: first, the availability of niacin in the digestive tract was found to be affected by the method of cooking; second, a sparing action on the amount of niacin was found with the amino acid tryptophan occurring in proteins. These problems were eventually resolved by the discovery that in such materials as corn, some niacin is bound in a form difficult to utilize. Also, tryptophan, when it is very plentiful, was found to serve as a precursor for part of the body's requirement for niacin.

Here culture again plays a part in nutrition. New World Indians of the south grew a lot of corn and had reasonably good nutrition, eating the corn along with certain other items such as legumes. The secret was that they had learned to store the corn in the ground with alkali for the long winter months. This product was good for them. By treating the corn with alkali under these conditions they released the bound or poorly utilizable nicotinic acid and made the tryptophan easier to use. Some people have stated that when corn was introduced into southern Europe, the Europeans took the product but not the culture. Corn was not treated under conditions to make the nutrients more available, and in some areas pellagra developed when corn was the main food.

During the 1930s, and even up until the late 1940s, many advances in nutrition occurred, particularly regarding the discovery and identification of different vitamins and their functions. As a result, vitamins could be added to research diets in order to learn how to balance the diet for general use and optimal nutrition. Fortunately, much of this knowledge was available before World War II and was introduced as public health concepts, e.g., vitamin fortification.

With all the information available on nutrition today, it is possible to design a nutritionally adequate diet. But even now there are some fads and fancies in nutrition, differences of opinion, and certainly comparatively large differences in the lifestyles of individuals, all of which have a bearing on what food is eaten. Someone sitting before a word processor all day and a television in the evening would have a greatly lower caloric requirement than someone leading an expedition to climb Mt. Everest. Usually, sedentary occupations and activities require 1,600 to 2,200 kilocalories of energy, while the climber of Mt. Everest would require over 4,000, and perhaps even as much as 5,000. But as calories go up, some of the other minor constituents of the foodstuffs, such as vitamins, may also need to increase to enable proper utilization of the increased calories.

Calories come from the main constituents of foodstuffs: proteins, carbohydrates and fats, with fats the greatest contributor. We have already read about the Indian high-fat food preparation, pemmican, which contained as much as 60% fat by weight. This supplies over 80% of the calories as fat! To many of us such a diet would seem nauseating, but to men carrying heavy packs up and down rough terrain for many miles a day, the energy given by these diets was undoubtedly welcomed. Today some of the recommendations for diets in more developed countries are for 30% or less calories as fat in the diet.

Still another consideration regarding the macrodietary constituents is the matter of bulk, and the type of bulk. For many years seamen and explorers knew that a completely refined diet was not a healthful one, and they resorted to the inclusion of materials like oatmeal and dried fruits. Today we are not only concerned about these for their general effect on daily health, such as relief of constipation, but also for their possible effects on carcinogenicity. The general thought today is that it is desirable to include fiber in the diet in order to maintain a healthy lower intestinal system.

Of course, it is not just a matter of having a balance of carbohydrates, proteins, fat and fiber, but also the inclusion of substances that we know to be essential, sometimes in large and sometimes in very minute amounts, that is important. The main items needed in larger amounts are the amino acids in proteins. Proteins differ greatly in their contents of the twenty or so recognized amino acids, and the requirement for some of these amino acids is now well known. Other amino acids are called unessential and can be synthesized by the biochemical system of the body. This is why there are good and poor proteins. One very poor protein preparation was the potable soup that was used extensively aboard British man-of-war ships two centuries ago. This was made from the hoofs and other discarded parts of animals and was almost devoid of some of the essential amino acids. Happily, some proteins are high in some essential amino acids and low in others, while other proteins may have the reverse combination of essential amino acids. Therefore, a diet including a mixture of such proteins would be important. A famous experiment in animal husbandry was done at the University of Wisconsin in the early 1900s in which the experimenters fed farm animals single grains and found that they did very poorly. When they mixed different grains, the animals did well, thus showing from a very practical standpoint the presence of important constituents in each of the grains that were lacking or low in others. So when a nutritionist talks about a balanced diet, more is meant than merely a balance of fruits, vegetables and so forth, as it should also include the proper mixture of different substances.

An obvious question frequently asked is why some amino acids are essential and others are not. The answer is a simple one: man is not capable of synthesizing the ones that are essential to him. Of course all the twenty recognized amino acids are essential to him, but the ones termed essential are the ones the body cannot synthesize from other amino acids or other protein sources. This same synthetic requirement also fits materials such as the vitamins, which are required in much lower, sometimes even tiny, amounts. If man could synthesize the vitamins then they would not be needed in his diet, but since he cannot, they must be included. There are some exceptions, such as when partial synthesis occurs, but this may not provide enough. Minerals and salts required in the diet are, of course, all essential; they're essential because they're needed, but also because man is incapable of their synthesis.

Before going into a further discussion of vitamins, perhaps an insight into essentiality is best provided. Fundamental research on the metabolism of cells has shown that even simple cellular organisms require many of the amino acids and catalysts that man needs. (If the catalyst cannot be synthesized by the organism, then it is usually called a vitamin.) Some bacteria not only require all those amino acids necessary in the diet of man but additional ones as well, and their requirements for many of the B vitamins may be equally as stringent. For this reason some bacteria are used as assay organisms to determine the amount of B vitamins in foodstuffs.

My introduction to basic nutrition was actually through bacterial nutrition when, as a graduate student at the University of Wisconsin, I did research on the development of bacterial methods for the determination of B vitamins. This interest in nutritional requirements of bacteria was continued, but with a different objective, in work as a lowly staff member at Harvard Medical School, where the research was to determine the nutritional requirements for the growth of a pathogenic organism, the tetanus bacillis (*Clostridium tetani*), in order to help produce its toxins which are used to manufacture injectable toxoids for medical use. Here other interrelationships were found to be critical, in that there was an optimal amount of iron necessary for the bacteria to make toxin; too little iron, no growth, and too much iron, no toxin. Further work with which I was later associated was in the opposite direction of requirements, with an organism called *Bacillus subtilis*. Here my colleagues and I showed that the requirements were extremely simple and devoid of all essential amino acids and vitamins. All that was necessary for this organism was a supply of energy, that is, carbohydrate, and then nitrogen as ammonia and salts. The organism was completely capable of synthesizing all the vitamins and all the amino acids. Now here again there was a sensitivity to the organism's requirements for a particular function, in this case the formation of an antibiotic named subtilin. Under conditions where good growth was obtained, not much antibiotic formation could occur.

Such differences with these minute living organisms should make it easier to explain why differences occur in much more complicated species, man and other animals. For example, man requires vitamin C, while many other animals do not. Luckily, the guinea pig was early found to require vitamin C, so an assay was available. The common experimental animal, the laboratory rat, does not require vitamin C, but hundreds of years ago sailors knew that rats made good food on long voyages. According to different stories, some ship captains fed cooked rats to themselves and some sailors, while in other cases the men in charge of the lower decks had a monopoly on the rat population and cooked and sold them to fellow mates. Luckily the rat is one of the greatest synthesizers of vitamin C. In contrast, man lacks a critical enzyme required in the synthetic sequence for making vitamin C. Thus, for man this compound is a vitamin; for the rat it is not.

For any animal, its physiological processes can alter its nutritional requirements. A vitamin that has a particular requirement for some is vitamin B_{12}. This vitamin was early known as a growth requirement in bacteria and only later shown to be the vitamin involved in a once very serious disease in humans, pernicious anemia. In this disease there is an essential substance in the stomach, called an intrinsic factor, which is required to complex the vitamin B_{12} that is eaten in the diet, and this complex is then properly assimilated in the digestive system. In those individuals with pernicious anemia, the intrinsic factor secretion in the stomach is very low or absent, so the vitamin B_{12}, although present in adequate amounts in the diet, is not utilized. Today this disease is rather well controlled by injections of vitamin B_{12}, which can then be directly used. Still another such interrelationship is involved in the fat-soluble vitamin,

vitamin D. Vitamin D is normally synthesized in the skin of humans when they are exposed to enough ultraviolet irradiation. As a consequence, people with little or no exposure to the sun have a much higher need for vitamin D in the diet than those who do have the exposure. These are just two of many examples of the complications that are found in maintaining good nutritional health.

Other important biological substances are nucleic acids and their constituent purines and pyrimidines. Some microorganisms require purines and pyrimidines, but humans do not. This may be a fortunate evolutionary consequence, because nucleic acids are the stuff that is in genes. Nutritional deficiencies of them would mean less opportunity, perhaps, to influence the genetic process in procreation. This is the case despite the belief of some individuals that eating animal glands, such as sweetbreads, would increase their sexual vigor.

As mentioned previously, foodstuffs and their requirements may be divided into macro and micro substances. This applies both to minerals and salts as well as to vitamins. Table A-1 lists the names of some of the important required nutrients. Some overlap is present in what is considered their function, or, in some cases, in the symptoms that are seen due to deficiencies. These are not necessarily the same, although usually related. Table A-2 lists the names and requirements of the principal vitamins and trace elements. Some of the vitamins are seldom, if ever, absent from a reasonably normal diet, although "reasonably normal" is a broad, and perhaps meaningless, term when comparing diets around the world or under certain stringent conditions. But the reason for the differences in requirements is that many living things produce enough of the vitamins to meet man's requirements, if even only small amounts are eaten. As a consequence, nutritional deficiencies in some of the vitamins, such as pantothenic acid, are very seldom seen. On the other hand, diseases like beriberi, pellagra, or hypovitaminosis A are frequently seen. In fact, hypovitaminosis A is endemic in many of the third world countries where serious ophthalmic problems are found in a large number of infants.

Before 1930 in the United States very few people, if anyone, took anything resembling vitamin tablets. Cod liver oil was used and yeast tablets were recommended. Cod liver oil provided both vitamins A and D, and the yeast tablets, a plethora of B vitamins, which was very fortunate. Even yeast tablets were eschewed by some physicians, and yeast cakes made from fresh yeast cells were recommended. In many cases these recommendations probably did the job very well. Today the manufacture of vitamin

Table A-1

U.S. recommended daily dietary allowances[a]

	Age (Years)	Weight (kg)	Weight (lb)	Height (cm)	Height (in)	Protein (g)	Fat-soluble Vitamins Vitamin A (µg R.E.)[b]	Fat-soluble Vitamins Vitamin D (mg)[c]	Fat-soluble Vitamins Vitamin E (mg a T.E.)[d]
Infants	0.0–0.5	6	13	60	24	kg x 2.2	420	10	3
	0.5–1.0	9	20	71	28	kg x 2.0	400	10	4
Children	1–3	13	29	90	35	23	400	10	5
	4–6	20	44	112	44	30	500	10	6
	7–10	28	62	132	52	34	700	10	7
Males	11–14	45	99	157	62	45	1,000	10	8
	15–18	66	145	176	69	56	1,000	10	10
	19–22	70	154	177	70	56	1,000	7.5	10
	23–50	70	154	178	70	56	1,000	5	10
	51+	70	154	178	70	56	1,000	5	10
Females	11–14	46	101	157	62	46	800	10	8
	15–18	55	120	163	64	46	800	10	8
	19–22	55	120	163	64	44	800	7.5	8
	23–50	55	120	163	64	44	800	5	8
	51+	55	120	163	64	44	800	5	8
Pregnant						+30	+200	+5	+2
Lactating						+20	+400	+5	+3

a. The allowances are intended to provide for individual variations among most normal persons living in the United States under usual environmental stresses. Diets should be based on a variety of common foods in order to provide other nutrients for which human requirements have been less well defined.

b. Retinol equivalents. 1 Retinol equivalent = 1 µg retinol or 6 µg ß carotene

c. As cholecalciferol. 10mg cholecalciferol = 400 I.U. vitamin D.

d. A tocopherol equivalents (T.E.). 1 mg d-∝-tocopherol = 1 a T.E.

Table A-2

Estimated safe and adequate daily dietary intakes of additional selected vitamins and minerals[a]

	Age (years)	Vitamins			Trace Elements[b]	
		Vitamin K (µg)	Biotin (µg)	Pantothenic Acid (mg)	Copper (mg)	Manganese (mg)
Infants	0–0.5	12	35	2	0.5–0.7	0.5–0.7
	0.5–1	10–20	50	3	0.7–1.0	0.7–1.0
Children and	1–3	15–30	65	3	1.0–1.5	1.0–1.5
Adolescents	4–6	20–40	85	3–4	1.5–2.0	1.5–2.0
	7–10	30–60	120	4–5	2.0–2.5	2.0–3.0
	11+	50–100	100–200	4–7	2.0–3.0	2.5–5.0
Adults		70–140	100–200	4–7	2.0–3.0	2.5–5.0

a. Because there is less information on which to base allowances, these figures are not given in the main table of the RDA and are provided here in the form of ranges of recommended intakes.

b. Since the toxic levels for many trace elements may be only several times usual intakes, the upper levels for the trace elements given in this table should not be habitually exceeded.

and megavitamin supplements is a huge industry, although how much of these supplements are really needed is frequently questioned. Furthermore, *megavitamin* supplementation can actually cause serious medical problems. Large amounts of both vitamins A and D, for example, are well known to cause clinical pathology in man, as seen in the discussion of the Eskimo diet and the toxicities that occurred when dog liver was eaten during the famous expedition of Douglas Mawson. This will be discussed further in appendix C. Then there are some megadoses that many tolerate well. With vitamin C, exceedingly large doses (as much as 10 grams per day, over 100-fold the recommended daily requirement) for the prevention of colds and viruses have been recommended by Dr. Linus Pauling. Nevertheless, good nutrition is attained with an optimal balance of dietary constituents.

appendix b
Food and Nutrition in the Frozen Cold

To most people living in the northernmost regions of the world, some items in their food menu were frequently frozen, and sometimes not even thawed. Practical experiences taught that some changes in food might result from freezing. Perhaps the dairy scientists studying ice cream were among the earliest applying rigorous scientific methods to study changes caused by freezing. Only during the last half century, however, has there been a concerted scientifically based effort to understand the properties, good and bad, of frozen foods. Even these studies have been primarily addressing the physical properties, which have a high impact on the sales of foods. Flavor, taste, and odor have been the main important characteristics.

In contrast to the efforts devoted to the above properties are those lesser ones that have been given to the properties related to nutrition. Most of this comparative lack of attention to the nutritional values of frozen foods probably stems from the long-time successful usage of frozen foods in practice as well as a few limited studies on their nutritional values.

When it comes to studies on the nutrition of people in frozen climates, even less information is available. As are studies on nutritional values of frozen foods, studies on human nutrition in frozen climates are limited and much of the work is by the military. Again, practical experiences over many centuries do not seem to have shown any unusual requirements, except possibly for a requirement of more calories.

The process of freezing food is the process of freezing water, although the constituents of each different food substance may affect the process in different ways. How water turns to its crystalline solid form, ice, has been studied by many of the world's finest scientists. Well over a century ago Michael Faraday and John Tyndall realized the importance of the freezing action. Tyndall's classic book, *The Forms of Water in Clouds, Rivers, Ice and*

Glaciers,[1] cites their questions, such as, How, when two blocks of ice were placed next to one another, do they become a single block of ice? Today many studies are published monthly on ice and the freezing process. Hobbs' book, *Ice Physics,* is an excellent source for insights into the physics of ice.[2]

Freezing for food preservation was used in prehistoric times. When a food was frozen hard, that was all that mattered, even up to the first part of the 20th century. Then, with the start of using mechanical refrigeration, freezing rooms were constructed. Soon these were displaced by separate freezing rooms, usually at less than -15°C, and storage rooms usually at -5° to -10°C. Now there are special temperatures for both freezing and storage depending upon the food product.

Freezing has been primarily used to inhibit microbial growths and their attendant undesirable effects. Both molds and bacteria have their growth inhibited and in most instances their viability impaired, but freezing is not a method for killing all of the bacteria. To emphasize this important safety matter, freezing does not sterilize foods.

During frozen storage chemical reactions may occur, some classified as enzymatic (catalytic) (table B-1) and others nonenzymatic (table B-2). Over longer periods, these reactions can usually make the food less palatable.

In addition to the actual freezing of a food, both the ways that foods are stored after freezing and the ways that they are thawed have a major effect on their qualities. On frozen storage, a change of crystal structure of the ice may occur, causing many small crystals to disappear and form much larger crystals of ice. This is called recrystallization. Recrystallization frequently occurs as a food is slowly thawed. Sometimes this may only cause a gritty effect as is sometimes found in ice cream stored in a home refrigerator. Other times, as with frozen organs, more undesirable physical changes of the tissue can be caused by the large crystals on recrystallization.

Because water is the major component of most foods and each food has its own particular water content, as well as its own particular structure, freezing processes for different foods may need to be specially tailored. Some foods such as juices can be frozen without any pretreatment and can be frozen by a variety of means. Other fluids like egg yolk develop a jelly-like consistency unless high concentrations of sugar are added. Still others, like some vegetables, must be rapidly frozen to prevent damage. Sometimes, the product may separate into several phases, becoming watery. Obviously, early explorers consumed many frozen foods that had lost their quality from freezing, frozen storage, and thawing.

Table B-1
Examples of nonenzymatic reactions that can accelerate in foods during freezing[a]

Type of reaction	Substrate
Acid-catalyzed hydrolysis	Sucrose
Oxidation	Ascorbic acid
	Butterfat
	Lipids in cooked beef
	Tocopherol in fried potato products
	ß–Carotene and vitamin A in fat
	Tuna and beef oxymyoglobin
	Milk
Protein insolubilization	Beef, rabbit, and fish protein
Formation of nitric oxide myoglobin or hemoglobin (cured meat color)	Myoglobin or hemoglobin

a. Adapted from O. Fennema, *Proteins at Low Temperature, Advances in Chemistry Series No. 180* (Washington, D.C.: American Chemical Society, 1979).

Table B-2
Some instances in which cellular systems exhibit increased rates of enzyme-catalyzed reactions during freezing[a]

Type of reaction	Sample	Temperature (°C) at which increased reaction rate was observed
Glycogen loss and/or accumulation of lactic acid	Frog, fish, beef, or poultry muscle	-2.5 to -6
Degradation of high energy phosphates	Fish, beef, and poultry muscle	-2 to -8
Hydrolysis of phospholipids	Cod	-4 (T_{max})
Decomposition of peroxides	Catalase in rapidly frozen potatoes and slowly frozen peas	-0.8 to -5
Oxidation of L-ascorbic acid	Rose hips, strawberries, Brussels sprouts	-10 -6 -2.5 to -5

a. Adapted from O. Fennema, *Proteins at Low Temperature, Advances in Chemistry Series No. 180* (Washington, D.C.: American Chemical Society, 1979).

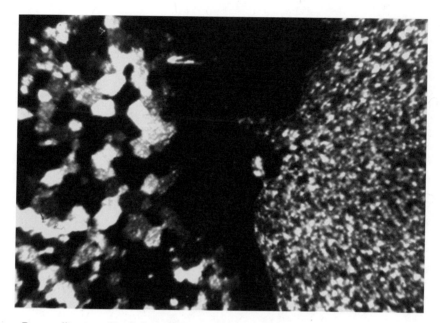

Recrystallization of ice from small crystals to large ones on frozen storage. Water is on the left. Inhibition by proteins from antarctic fish blood is on the right.
Yeh and Feeney, 1996

Surveying the animal kingdom, humans may be placed as tropical animals.[3] How have they been able to live in the coldest areas of the earth? Some possibilities could include an inherited special cold resistant physiology or the consumption of special foods. Neither of these appears true. Other than some minor physical characteristics that might make cold living easier, people like Eskimos more likely just learned how to adapt and adjust their physiology to their cold environment.

The normal human body temperature of 37°C is carefully maintained by a variety of physiological safeguards. Should the body temperature begin to drop, the brain begins to slow down and all sorts of unpleasant results occur, such as poor coordination, confusion, and apathy. In turn, these can cause the individual to become careless about protecting himself from the cold and have accidents. Finally, on reaching a temperature much below 34°C, he will soon become comatose and then die. Poor physical fitness, physical injury, or caloric deficit can cause a body to drop below a level of metabolism critical for maintaining energy and heat production. Providing a palatable diet of sufficient calories is a major challenge for cold weather nutrition.[4]

As with many other studies that the military groups have conducted, cold weather physiology and nutrition have been areas where the militaries have done the primary work. Not surprisingly, the cold war of the last half of the 20th century supplied stimuli for studies in cold regions.[5] Reviews on activities in cold environments more generally emphasize physiology.[6]

Because of the numerous worldwide nutritional deficiencies, sufficient calories are still a significantly important need for people in warmer environments as well as in the cold. To polar explorers, sufficient energy in the diet was frequently a critical need. Askew has summarized the need for energy in the cold.

> There are numerous factors that influence energy intake and expenditure in cold environments. Energy requirements are influenced by the intensity of the cold, wind speed, difficulty of working under winter conditions (achieving shelter, melting snow, traveling on difficult surfaces, etc.), and the light-dark cycle (in arctic areas) (Henschell, 1960; Campbell, 1982). At the same time that energy requirements are high, energy intakes may be reduced by factors such as the monotony of the diet (lack of locally available foodstuffs) and the difficulty of preparing food for consumption under adverse conditions.[7]

Table B-3
Energy expenditure for typical cold weather military activities[a]

Activity[b]	Energy Expenditure (kcal/min)
Sleeping (tent, sleeping bag)	1.3
Leisure activities in tent (2°C)	1.8
Trail marching (30 kg pack, weapon)	4.8
Sledge hauling (3 man team, 170 kg sledge)	8.6–10.4
Daily energy expenditure	**(kcal/day)**
Bivouac	2665
Patrol	3300–3600
Average for 2 week arctic exercise	3250
Average body weight loss/2 week	1.0 kg

a. From W. J. O'Hara, C. Allen, and R. J. Shepard, "Loss of Body Fat During An Arctic Winter Expedition," *Canadian Journal of Physiological Pharmacology* 55 (1977): 1235–1241.
b. Data collected on Canadian infantrymen in the vicinity of Ft. Churchill, Manitoba, and Baffin Island, N.W.T. Temperatures averaged -23°C.

Table B-4

Details of energy balance measurements made on sledging journeys[a]

Authors	Mode of travel	n	Duration of journey (d)	Mean energy intake (kcal)	Method of measure-ment	Estimated energy expenditure (kcal)	Mean body weight (kg)	Weight change (kg)
Masterson, et. al (1957)	Dog sledge	2	19	4660	Inference[b]	5065	73.5	—
	Dog sledge	2	10	4850	Inference	5330	85	—
Norman (1965)	Manhauling	4	7	4420	Individual weighing	5045	79.5	-1.25
Orr (1965)	Dog sledge	2	19	3895	Inference	—	76	-2.25
	Dog sledge	2	13	4085	Inference	—	79.5	-1.75
	Dog sledge	3	70	4995	Inference	—	71	0
	Dog sledge	3	18	5590	Inference	—	84	0
Acheson (1974)	Dog sledge	2	21	3155	Individual weighing	3250	71.2	-1.7
	Manhauling	2	7	3320	Individual weighing	4085	70.1	-1.6
Campbell (1975)	Dog sledge	2	19	2560	Individual weighing	3990	78.5	-1.7
	Motor sledge	2	14	2365	Individual weighing	2870	64	-1.5
	Manhauling	2	20	3050	Individual weighing	3895	64.2	-1.6
Boyd (1975)	Motor sledge	3	42	4040	Inference	3490	76.2	-6.2
Campbell (1981)	Manhauling	6	37	3945	Individual weighing	—	77.8	-2.3

a. From I. T. Campbell,1982. "Nutrition in adverse environments," and "Energy balance under polar conditions," *Human Nutrition: Applied Nutrition* 36A (1982): 196–178.

b. Inference: Energy intakes were inferred from the known energy contents of food boxes.

Much higher energy was found to be expended in man-hauling sledges as compared to trail-marching (with 30 kg pack and weapon) (table B-3). With dog sledge the caloric requirements, perhaps depending upon the amounts of riding, walking, or pushing (table B-4) are less, but they could be equally as high. According to Askew, caloric demands for moderate to high activity in arctic and subarctic areas are usually adequately supported by 4,000–5,000 kcal/man/day.

Not everything, however, is related to calories. Older naval nonpolar as well as polar explorations were usually associated with scurvy. Certainly a diet balanced in vitamins, minerals, and proteins is necessary, and sufficient consumption of water is also critical. And just the cold itself has many effects. Even breathing in cold air can be hazardous. As measured by endurance times on exposure of men heavily clothed, those at +20°C had twice the endurance time of those at -20°C.[8] During my times working in Antarctica, I encountered a number of different adjustments to the food supplied.[9] At the main base of McMurdo, Ross Island, with meals available four times a day, some men consumed too many calories and grew fat. Other men were able to obtain food from the supplies and do most of their own cooking as small groups, possibly not selecting a balanced diet.[10] Coming into a warm tent from working at low temperatures during blizzards, I also drank too much hot coffee and not enough water until I became dehydrated.

Probably it is not correct in this short discussion to offer definite conclusions on cold nutrition. Various articles cited here could be consulted. Research on the effects of unbalanced diets, like ketogenic ones, is still in progress.

Notes

1. J. Tyndall, *The Forms of Water in Clouds and Rivers, Ice, and Glaciers* (New York: D. Appleton and Co., 1896), 163.
2. P. V. Hobbs, *Ice Physics*, (Oxford: Oxford University Press, 1974).
3. L. D. Carlson and A. C. L. Hsieh, "Cold," in *The Physiology of Human Survival*, O. G. Edhom and A. L. Bacharach, ed. (London: Academic Press, 1965), 15.
4. E. W. Askew, LTC, "Nutrition and Performance in Cold Environments," 40th Annual Meeting of Research and Development Associates for Military Food and Packaging, Inc., Orlando, Florida (1986).
5. Askew, "Nutrition and Performance in Cold Environments." See also, H. E. Lewis, "Nutritional Research in the Polar Regions," *Nutrition Reviews* 21 (1963): 353–356.
6. L. D. Carlson and A.C. L. Hsieh, 15. See also E. M. Haymes and C. L. Wells, ed., "Cold Environments and Human Performance," in *Environment and Human Performance* (Champaign, Illinois: Human Kinetics Publishers, Inc., 1986), 43–68;

S. D. Phinney et al., "The Human Response to Chronic Ketosis without Caloric Restrictions: Preservation of Submaximal Exercise Capabilities with Reduced Carbohydrate Oxidation," *Metabolism* 32, 8 (1983): 769.

7. E. W. Askew, "Nutrition and Performance in Cold Environments," 40th Annual Meeting of Research and Development Associates for Military Food and Packaging, Inc., Orlando, Florida, 1986, page 2.

8. J. F. Patton and J. A. Vogel, "Effects of Cold Exposure on Submaximal Endurance Performance," *Med. Sci. Sports, Exerc* 16 (1984): 494–497.

9. R. E. Feeney, *Professor on the Ice* (Davis: Pacific Portals, 1974).

10. While spending several weeks in a tent at Cape Crozier in four different years, I gradually learned to like the eggs of Adelie penguins. Since then I have sometimes desired omelets made with chicken eggs and fish, because the bird's diet of ocean items made the penguin eggs taste fishy. Boiled eggs, however, were not as appetizing. As duck eggs do on boiling, penguin eggs gave glassy whites. Cracked penguin's eggs were available from our work with the nearly half-million birds nesting at Cape Crozier.

appendix c
Hypervitaminosis A

A s with many other essential nutrients, very high levels of vitamin A cannot be tolerated by man, or by many other animals. Fortunately, with vitamin A there is a very great difference between the requirement for the vitamin and the higher level causing toxicity. In spite of this rather wide safety range, hypervitaminosis A has most likely occurred in both polar areas. Certainly it now occurs in the general population when individuals, for various reasons, dose themselves with high levels of vitamin A.

Hypervitaminosis in Eskimos

Numerous scattered reports indicate that Eskimos avoid eating polar bear, husky dog, and seal livers. Although there are some differences of opinion among various workers, the review by David Landy includes a general discussion of possible hypervitaminosis A in an Eskimo people (the Inuit). The review is particularly related to what has been termed *pibloktoq* (hysteria).[1]

We will not challenge the numerous statements that Eskimos in most cases avoid eating polar bear, husky dog, and some other livers. Although there are also numerous examples where they do eat these livers, perhaps in most of these instances only small amounts of liver were eaten. In addition, as is discussed further in this book, the nutritional status of the individual, as well as what other items are being consumed with the liver, may influence the toxicity.

To Inuit, *pibloktoq* is an abnormal state that may affect anyone. According to Landy the term *pibloktoq* refers to a hysterical reaction among the people, and it is one of a group of aberrant behaviors occurring among arctic and circumarctic societies. It is sometimes called arctic hysteria and has been explained by many different theories based on "ecological, nutritional, biological, physiological, psychological, psychoanalytic, social structure, and cultural factors."[2] In Landy's article he suggests that *pibloktoq* may, in some instances, be a result of vitamin intoxication, that is, hypervitaminosis A. He supports a multifactorial framework in which a number of causes may operate simultaneously, including in some instances hypervitaminosis A. There may be several causes that are not mutually exclusive, and two or more of them may interact with one another. He cites a description of *pibloktoq* as made by A. Wallace:

> (1) Prodrome: the individual may be irritable or withdrawn for hours or a day; (2) excitement: suddenly, without much warning, the victim becomes wildly excited and may perform many irrational acts, frequently running out of the shelter and having to be rescued; (3) convulsions and stupor: the excitement is followed by convulsive seizures and by collapse; (4) recovery: the individual may now behave normally and even state he does not remember what happened.[3]

The disease appears to also be found in dogs, where it is called *piblokto*. When a pack had this, many would be affected. The disease did not appear to be related to any known dog disease at that time.

Although the general clinical picture of *pibloktoq* does not equate with other symptoms of hypervitaminosis A, such as loss of skin and hair, the interpretation of Landy's conclusions is that perhaps a milder form of the toxicity, such as would be obtained by eating high quantities of the body fat of seals or polar bears together with some entrails, might be a contributing factor along with other clinical problems. These other problems could be the otitis media, which was chronic among some Eskimos, some malnutrition, and some psychologically based diseases.

There are apparently no satisfactory records showing that Eskimos ate polar bear liver in any quantities that might cause severe hypervitaminosis A. Perhaps under extreme conditions, where a group might have to resort to eating their husky dogs, if the liver were consumed it would be divided among enough individuals so that the quantity would be insufficient to cause recognizable symptoms. It is also possible that the taboos were so strong that there are few examples to cite.

Buried here and there, probably some fact and some fable, are statements that arctic explorers were ill affected by eating bear liver. Several reports, however, appear well described and must be considered true.

In Barent's expedition to Novaya Zemlya in 1596, many members became quite ill after eating bear liver. Three became very ill and lost their skin from head to foot.[4]

The explorer E. K. Kane experimented with eating bear liver and found that poisoning did not always occur. Sometimes there were no ill effects in his company of men, but on two occasions the entire company became sick after eating bear liver.[5]

Still later members of the English expedition to Franz Joseph Land in 1894–1897 (part of the group that rescued Nansen) ate polar bear liver and they all became ill. In this instance they were served by Koettlitz, a physician (who was Scott's physician in Antarctica).[6]

Even in the early 20th century, cases were reported in the Arctic. According to Lindhard nineteen men of a group who consumed a stew made from the liver, heart and kidneys of one large bear all became sick.[7] Several victims became ill within four hours of the meal and the rest during the night. They appeared to have the usual symptoms of food poisoning: irritability, severe headache and vomiting, etc. By the second day the skin of ten of the nineteen patients began to peel. In other instances Lindhard found that in three cases the skin peeled from head to foot after eating bear liver.

Research and Clinical Evidence for Hypervitaminosis A Toxicity

One of the earliest studies suggesting that the high vitamin A content in liver might be toxic if eaten in even small amounts was done by Takashi and coworkers.[8] Perhaps one of the classical publications was by K. Rodahl and T. Moore.[9] In their paper, "The vitamin A content and toxicity of bear and seal liver," they described analyses of bear livers for vitamin A and experiments in feeding rats. Values for vitamin A in the three different specimens varied from 13,000 I.U. per gram to 18,000 I.U. per gram of wet material. (One I.U., the International Unit, is equivalent to 0.3 microgram of pure vitamin A.) In the rats they found the livers to be highly toxic, producing skin lesions, ruffling and the loss of hair, peeling of the skin, and then the onset of other diseases such as enteritis, emaciation, and pneumonia. In attempting to extrapolate their rat results to humans, they estimated that it would take about 7,500,000 I.U. (or 2.5 grams of pure vitamin A) to cause illness in a 70 kg man. This amount would be present in 375 grams (a little over three-quarters of a pound) of bear liver, which was not considered an excessive portion.

As a consequence of such toxicity reports, as well as interest in possible sources of vitamin A, there have been many analyses of livers for vitamin A content. It is well known that some marine species have high contents and, indeed, this is possibly why the polar bear accumulates so much vitamin A

Table C-1

Typical values for the hepatic reserves of vitamin A in different species[a]

Species	Vitamin A[b] I.U./g liver	Species	Vitamin A I.U./g liver
Guinea pig	10	Horse	600
Frog	30	Hen	900
Pig	100	Greenland seal	2,000
Dog[c]	100	Cod fish	2,000
Vole	100	Python	3,000
Cow	150	Giant monitor	4,000
Rabbit	150	Sperm whale	4,500
Rat	250	Halibut	10,000
Human	300	Bearded seal	13,000
Fox	500	Polar bear	20,000
Sheep	600		

a. In every species wide individual variations are to be expected.
b. Given as International Units. 1 I.U. = 0.3 of vitamin A retinol equivalents.
c. Polar dogs have very much higher amounts of Vitamin A.
Source: T. Moore, *Vitamin A* (Amsterdam: Elsevier, 1957).

in his liver as a result of eating fish. Table C-1 shows the vitamin A contents in international units (I.U.) per gram, all the way from as low as ten in guinea pigs to as high as 50,000 in the shark fin soup. Polar bear was near the top of the list, but even with these results there is still a question as to the presence of other toxic materials accumulating in the liver.

General Scientific Evidence for Toxicity of Hypervitaminosis A

When the toxicities from eating the livers of arctic animals such as polar bears and husky dogs are considered, it is necessary to go back to their diets of marine species and high fat. Yoshiro Hashimoto, in his book *Marine Toxins and Other Bioactive Marine Metabolites*, has a section entitled "Hypervitaminosis A Caused by Fish Liver."[10] He cites old records in Japan, dating back to the 1880s, that reported poisoning when livers of some larger fish, such as sharks, tunas and sea bass, were eaten. In 1960 marketing of sea bass liver was prohibited, but poisoning still occurred sporadically, even with that ban. The livers of old fish contained even much higher amounts of vitamin A, irrespective of the fish species. The disease was described as *ichthyohepatotoxism*. In sixteen cases the most characteristic symptom was desquamation, which appeared a few days after ingestion. In severe cases this extended over the entire body, and large areas of skin peeled. However, Hashimoto has a note of caution in his discussion, stating that there may be also other toxic substances stored in the livers.

A comprehensive summary of vitamin A and nutrition, including both hypovitaminosis A and hypervitaminosis A, has been published in a report of the International Vitamin A Consultative Group by J. Christopher Baurenfeind, entitled "The Safe Use of Vitamin A."[11] For detailed information on the subject, this report should be consulted. Vitamin A is described as an essential nutrient for man and as usually being supplied in the daily diet either as vitamin A, as carotenoid vitamin A precursors (such as found in carrots), or as a mixture of the two. When ingested in amounts greater than the daily need, it is stored in the liver. By far the greatest problem in the world is vitamin A deficiency, or hypovitaminosis A. Toxicity or hypervitaminosis A is much rarer because of the great difference between the requirement and the amount to cause toxicity.

The different stages in vitamin A nutrition have been described by Miller and Hayes and are traced in figure C-1.[12] A very low intake of vitamin A will eventually cause death. One of the great illnesses of the world in undeveloped countries is night blindness and xerophthalmia, with permanent blinding. It is estimated that there are over a million people afflicted annually worldwide, with 100,000 permanently blind. In a recommendation by the National Research Council for daily allowances as given in table C-2, for a grown man the requirement is 1,000 micrograms per day, or 3,300 I.U. per day. From the figure it can be seen that toxicity begins to occur at around 5,000–6,000 micrograms per kilogram of body weight per day, or around 400,000 micrograms per day for a 70 kilogram man. This gives a margin of safety of 350 times the recommended requirement. This is sometimes stated to be 1,000 times.

Hypervitaminosis A is divided into two categories: acute and chronic. It may occur in infants, children, and adults and may be caused by parents overdosing the children and by self-medication by individuals not understanding the danger. More likely than not, it exists in individuals who are health faddists and individuals not understanding the meaning of dosages and confusing such simple differences as drops and droppers full or drops and teaspoonsful. And then, of course, some have the idea that if a little is good, more would be better.

Even physicians themselves can overdose patients because of their honest beliefs that high dosages of vitamins are beneficial. Sometimes they

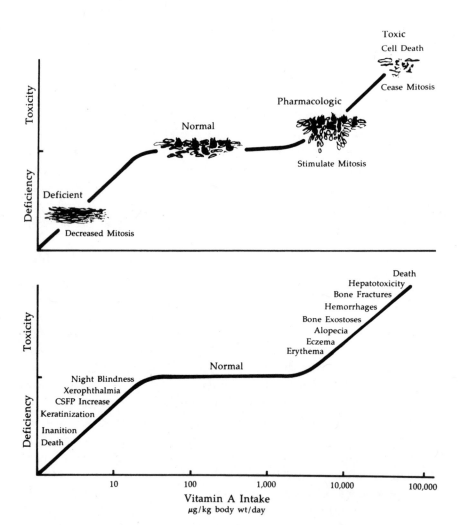

Figure C-1. The logarithmic plot of vitamin A intake is depicted as a function of the biological response of man and animals in terms of deficiency, normalcy, and toxicity. The scheme at the top illustrates the response of a typical mucous epithelium, but is probably applicable to other undifferentiated blast-cell populations as well. The bottom curve indicates the clinical manifestations resulting from the altered cell function in deficiency and toxicity of vitamin A. From J. C. Bauernfeind, 1980.

may give high doses to treat a particular disease but then continue it over too long a time. The patient may also continue the medication long after the physician thinks the treatment is finished because the patient can purchase the high-dosage vitamins himself. (Self-medication is probably encouraged by the advocates of the use of very high levels of ascorbic acid to prevent infections and even by the current recommendations of some physicians for the consumption of high levels of nicotinic acid to reduce the danger of cholesterol deposits in blood vessels.) Finally there are those cases, such as the ones we have already discussed, resulting from the consumption of polar bear, seal, walrus, husky dog, halibut, shark, and other animal livers.

Acute toxicity has apparently been seen in quite a number of cases where patients are treated for psoriasis. As much as 500,000 I.U. daily seem to be tolerated, but doses over 1,000,000 cause dryness, scaling, and fissuring of the lips, while 2,000,000 to 4,000,000 gives scaling of skin, nausea, and dizziness. In another case quoted by Baurenfeind, a 20-year-old man who had consumed 70 to 75 million I.U. of vitamin A over a 30-day period for treatment of psoriasis had extensive symptoms and was extremely ill with

Table C-2
FAO/WHO recommended daily allowance for vitamin A

Group	Age (years)	FAO/WHO Vitamin A Values (μg/day)[a]
Infants	0–1/2	(satisfied by breast feeding by well-nourished mother)
	1/2–1	300
Children	1	250
	2	250
	3	250
	4–6	300
	7–9	400
	10–12	575
	13–15[b]	725
	16–19[b]	750
Adults[c]	all ages	750

[a] To convert to I.U., multiply by 3.3.
[b] Boys and girls.
[c] Men and women.
Source: Baurenfeind, J.C., *The Safe Use of Vitamin A* (Report of the International Vitamin A Consultative Group), Office of Nutrition, Development Support Bureau, Agency for International Development, Department of State, Washington, D.C. (September 1980).

Table C-3
NRC recommended daily allowances for vitamin A

Group	Age (years)	Weight (lbs)	NRC-NAS Vitamin A Values (mg/day)[a]
Infants	0–1/2	13 (6)[b]	420
	1/2–1	20 (9)	400
Children	1–3	29 (13)	400
	4–6	44 (20)	500
	7–10	62 (28)	700
Males	11–14	99 (45)	1000
	19–22	145 (66)	1000
	23–50	154 (70)	1000
	51+	154 (70)	1000
Females	11–14	101 (46)	800
	15–18	120 (55)	800
	19–22	120 (55)	800
	23–50	120 (55)	800
	51+	120 (55)	800
Pregnant	—	—	1000
Lactating	—	—	1200

a. To convert to I.U., multiply by 3.3.
b. Weight in kg.
Source: Baurenfeind, J.C., *The Safe Use of Vitamin A* (Report of the International Vitamin A Consultive Group), Office of Nutrition, Development Support Bureau, Agency for International Development, Department of State, Washington, D.C. (September 1980).

all the textbook symptoms: headache, itching, vomiting, fatigue, anorexia, vertigo, painful extremities, reddening of the skin, gingivitis, ulcerated lips, renal tubular failure, and so forth. But after only twelve days cessation of the vitamin A treatment the patient recovered. In another case a woman ingested 1,300,000 I.U. over 27 hours in the belief that it would protect her from sunburn. She developed headache, nausea, skin exfoliation, and other symptoms. In infants and children acute hypervitaminoses occur quickly and show typical responses. In the very young there is a bulging of the fontanels following a single overdose of 300,000 to 900,000 I.U. When a twelve-year-old boy was administered an average of one million I.U. per day over 21 days for treatments of ichthyosis congenita, he developed severe headaches and loss of skin and other symptoms, beginning on the ninth day. The list goes on and on.

Chronic hypervitaminosis A is more common than one would think. In infants and young children it results in anorexia, dry and itchy skin, loss of hair, intracranial pressure, cracking of lips and other symptoms. In adults, milder joint and bone pains, but more skin and nail changes, as well as other toxic symptoms occur. In one classical case, a 21-year-old woman was admitted to five hospitals over nine years before her diagnosis as hypervitaminosis A was made in the sixth hospital. During most of the period she had been consuming 500,000 I.U. of vitamin A per day. Chronic hypervitaminosis A in children and infants is apparently something that should be watched more closely than it is.

The Case for Hypervitaminosis A in Polar Regions

All the experimental data in animals and the extensive data from patients are in direct agreement with what might be expected from eating large quantities of polar bear or husky dog livers. The general Eskimo taboo against consuming these livers thus seems in order, and most of the cases reported by explorers should be taken very seriously as being true. All of Mawson's symptoms, as well as those of his colleague, fall in line here. Nevertheless, other problems such as some scurvy, as well as other vitamin deficiencies, could also have contributed to their conditions, not wholly, but as an adjunctive effect contributing to the total pathology.

Notes

1. D. Landy, "Pibloktoq (Hysteria) and Inuit Nutrition: Possible Implication of Hypervitaminosis," *Soc. Sci. Med.* 21, 2 (1985): 173–185.
2. Ibid., 180.
3. A. F. C. Wallace, "Mental illness, biology, and culture," in *Psychological Anthropology*, F. L. K. Hsu (Cambridge: Shenkman, 1972), 363–402.
4. J. Richardson, *Polar Regions* (Edinborough: A. & B. Black, 1861), 71.
5. E. K. Kane, *Arctic Explorations. The Second Grinnell Expedition in Search of John Franklin, 1853, 1854, 1855* (Philadelphia: Childs and Peterson, 1856), 1392–1393.
6. R. Koettlitz, "Contributions to the Natural History of the Polar Bear (Ursus Maritimus, Linn.)," *Proc. Royal Physical Society* 14 (1898): 266–277.
7. J. Lindhard, "Health Conditions on the Danmark Expedition," *Medd Gronland* (1913): 457–468.
8. K. Takahashi, Z. Nazamiya, K. Kawakami, and T. Kitasato, "On the physical and chemical properties of Biosterin [a name given to fat-soluble A] and on its physiological significance," *Scientific Papers of the Institute of Physical and Chemical Research, Tokyo* 3 (1925): 81–146.

9. K. Rodahl and T. Moore, "The vitamin A content and toxicity of bear and seal liver," *Biochem. J.* 37 (1943): 166–168.

10. Y. Hashimoto, *Marine Toxins and Other Bioactive Marine Metabolites* (Tokyo: Japan Scientific Society's Press, 1979).

11. J. C Bauernfeind, *The Safe Use of Vitamin A*, Report of the International Vitamine A Consultative Group, Office of Nutrition, Development Support Bureau, Agency for International Development, Department of State, Washington, D.C. (September 1980).

12. D. R. Miller and K. C. Hayes, *Intake and Toxicity of Vitamins in Nutritional Toxicity*, J. N. Hathock, editor (New York: Academic Press, 1981): 160.

bibliography

Abraham, H. S. *Hero in Disgrace*. New York: Paragon House, 1971.

Adams, W. H. D. *Recent Polar Voyages: A Record of Discovery and Adventure, from Search after Franklin to the British Polar Expedition, 1875–1876*. London: Nelson and Sons, 1877.

Aigner, J. S. "Early Arctic Settlements in North America." *Scientific American* 253, 5 (1985): 160–169.

Alexandra, R. *Eskimo Cookbook*. Seattle: Hancock House Publishers, 1977.

Amundsen, R. *My Life as an Explorer*. Garden City: Doubleday, Page and Co., 1927.

———. *The Northwest Passage*. London: A. Constable and Co., 1908.

———. *The South Pole*. 2 vols. London: John Murray, 1913.

Amy, R.; R. Bhatnagar; E. Damkjar; and O. Beattie. "The Last Franklin Expedition: Report of a Postmortem Examination of a Crew Member." *Can. Med. Assoc. J* 135 (1986): 115–117.

Appert, N. *The Art of Preserving: Report of the Board of Arts and Manufacture*, Paris. Translated from the French. London: Black, Parry and Kingsbury, 1812.

Armstrong, A. *Observations on Naval Hygiene and Scurvy: More Particularily as the Latter Appeared During a Polar Voyage*. London: J. Churchill, 1858.

Askew, E. W., Lt.C. *Nutrition and Performance in Cold Environments*. 40th Annual Meeting of Research and Development Associates for Military. Orlando, Florida: Food and Packaging, Inc., 1986.

Balchen, B. "The Strange Enigma of Admiral Byrd." National Archives, Laurence Gould Collection, Correspondence, 1929–1971. RG 401(59), 1950.

Bandi, Hans-Georg. *Eskimo Prehistory*. Fairbanks: University of Alaska Press, 1969.

Bauernfeind, J. C. The Safe Use of Vitamin A. A Report of the International Vitamin A Consultative Group, Office of Nutrition, Development Support Bureau, Agency for International Development, Department of State. Washington, D. C., September 1980.

Beaglehole, J. C. *The Life of Captain James Cook*. Stanford: University Press, 1974.

247

Beardsley, T. "Down to Earth, Biosphere 2 Tries to Get Real." *Scientific American* 273, 2 (1995): 24–26.

Beattie, O., and J. Geiger. *Frozen in Time.* Saskatoon, Canada: Western Producer Prairie Books, 1987.

Beattie, O. B., and J. M. Savelle. "Discovery of Human Remains from Sir John Franklin's Last Expedition." *Historical Archaeology* 17, 2 (1983): 100–105.

Benedeit. See Short, I., and B. Merrilees, eds.

Bernstein, R. E. "Liver and hypervitaminosis." *New England Journal of Medicine* 311 (1984): 604–608.

Berton, P. *The Arctic Grail.* New York: Viking Penguin, 1988.

Bickel, L. *This Accursed Land.* Melbourne, Australia: Sun Books, 1978.

Binkerd, E. F.; O. E. Kolari; and C. Tracy. "Pemmican." *Maricopa Trails* 1, 1 (1977): 1–10.

Birket-Smith, Kaj. *The Eskimos,* 2nd edition. London: Methuen and Co., 1959.

Borchgrevink, C. E., *First on the Arctic Continent.* Montreal, Canada: McGill–Queen's University Press, 1962.

Borgstrom, G. *Food Technology.* Vol 1, *Principles of Food Science.* New York: MacMillan Co., 1968.

Bourland, C. T.; M. F. Fohey; V. L. Kloeris; and R. M. Rapp. "Designing a Food System for Space Station Freedom," *Food Technology* 43, 2 (1989): 76–81.

Breasted, J. H. "The Rise of Man." *Science* 74 (1931): 639–643.

Bryd, R. E. *Alone.* New York: G.M. Putnam's Sons, 1938.

Carlson, L.D., and A. C. L. Hsieh. In *The Physiology of Human Survival,* edited by O. G. Edhom and A. L. Bacharach. London: Academic Press, 1965.

Campbell, I. T. "Nutrition in adverse environments." *Human Nutrition: Applied Nutrition* 36A (1982): 196–178.

———. "Energy balance under polar conditions." *Human Nutrition: Applied Nutrition* 36A (1982): 196–178.

Carpenter, K. J. *The History of Scurvy and Vitamin C.* England: Cambridge University Press, 1986.

———. *Protein and Energy.* Cambridge, England: Cambridge University Press, 1994.

Carre, A. "Eighteenth-century French voyages of exploration: general problems of nutrition with special reference to the voyages of Bougainville and d'Entrecasteaux." In *Starving Sailors: The Influence of Nutrition upon Naval and Maritime History,* edited by J. Watt, E. J. Freeman, and W. F. Bynum. London: National Maritime Museum, 1981.

Cherry-Garrard, A. *The Worst Journey in the World.* London: Chatto and Windus Ltd., 1922.

Cleland, J., and R. V. Southcott. "Hypervitaminosis A in the Antarctic in the Australasian Antarctic Expedition of 1911–1914: A possible explanation of the illnesses of Mertz and Mawson." *Medical Journal of Australia* 1 (1969): 1337–1342

Conway, H. A., and A. I. Meyer, eds. *Ration Development.* Operations Studies Number 1, Volume 12. United States Armed Forces Quartermaster Food and Container Institute, 1947.

Cook, F. A. *My Attainment of the Pole.* New York : Lent and Griff, 1911.

———. *Return from the Pole.* New York: Pellegrini and Cudahy, 1951.

———. *Through the First Antarctic Night.* New York: Doubleday and McClure Co., 1900.

Cyriax, R. J. *Sir John Franklin's Last Arctic Expedition.* London: Methuen and Co., 1939.

Davies, T. D. "New Evidence Places Peary at the Pole." *National Geographic 177,* 1 (1990): 44.

Debenheim, F. *Discovery and Exploration.* London: Geographical Projects Limited, 1960.

DeLong, E., ed. *The Voyage of the Jeannette.* Vol. 1 and 2. Boston: Houghton, Mifflin Co., 1883.

Dennett, J. F. *The Voyages and Travels of Captains Ross, Parry, Franklin, and Mr. Belzoni.* London: William Wright, 1835.

Dickens, C. "The Lost Arctic Voyagers." *Household Words* 245 (December 2, 1854): 361–365.

Dodge, E. S. *Northwest by Sea.* New York: Oxford University Press, 1961.

Drummond, J. C. "The examination of some tinned foods of historic interest, part 1." *Chemistry and Industry* (August 27, 1938): 808–815.

Drummond, J. C., and W. R. Lewis. *The Examination of Some Tinned Foods of Historic Interest.* Intern. London: Tin Res. and Dev. Council, 1938.

Drummond, J. C., and A. Wilbraham. *The Englishman's Food of Sir Jack Drummond, Dec'd.* Oxford, England: Alder Press, 1958.

Ellis, H. A. *Voyage to Hudson's Bay by the Dobbs Galley and California in the Years 1746–1747.* London: Whitridge, 1748.

Evans, E.R.G.R. *South with Scott.* London: W. Collins Sons and Co., Ltd., 1921.

Falla, R. A. "Antarctic adventure and research." *New Zealand Sci. Review* 13 (1955): 107–116

Feeney, R. E. "Food technology and polar exploration." *Food Technology* 43, 5 (1989): 70, 72, 74, 76–82.

———. *Professor on the Ice.* Davis, Calif.: Pacific Portals, 1974.

———. *The World's Food Supply.* In *The Social Responsibility of the Scientist,* edited by M. Brown. New York: Free Press, 1971.

Feeney, R. E.; R. G. Allison; D. T. Osuga; J. C. Bigler; and H. T. Miller. Biochemistry of the Adelie Penquin: Studies on Egg and Blood Serum Proteins. *Antarctic Res. Series* 12. Reprinted from *Antarctic Bird Studies,* edited by J. R. Austin. American Geophysical Union., 1968.

Feeney, R. E.; E. L. Askew; and D. A. Jezior. "The Development and Evolution of U.S. Army Rations." *Nutrition Reviews* 53, 8 (1995): 221–225.

Feeney, R. E., and Y. Yeh. "Antifreeze Proteins: Properties, Mechanisms of Actions, and Possible Applications." *J. Food Technology* 47 (1993): 82–91.

Fennema, O. *Proteins at Low Temperature. Advances in Chemistry Series, No. 180.* Washington, D.C.: American Chemical Society, 1979.

Fiennes, Sir Ranulph. *To The Ends of the Earth. The Transglobal Expedition: the First Pole-to-Pole Circumnavigation of the Globe.* New York: Arbor House, 1983.

Fisher, V. *Pemmican.* Garden City, New York: Doubleday and Co., 1956.

Fogelson, Nancy. *Arctic Exploration and International Relations 1900–1932.* Fairbanks: University of Alaska Press, 1992.

Fogg, G. E. *A History of Antarctic Science.* Cambridge: Cambridge University Press.

Fortuine, Robert. "Scurvy and Its Influence on Early Alaskan History." *Arctic Medical Research Supplement 1,* 47 (1988).

Franklin, J. *Journey to the Shores of the Polar Sea in 1819–20–21–22.* London: John Murray, 1829.

Freedman, B. J. "Dr. Edward Wilson of the Antarctic. A Biographical sketch, followed by an inquiry into the nature of his last illness." *Proc. Royal Soc. Med., Section of the History of Medicine* 47 (1954): 183–189.

Freuchen, D., ed. *Peter Freuchen's Book of the Eskimos.* Cleveland, Ohio: World Publishing Co., 1961.

Fu, B., and P. E. Nelson. "Conditions and constraints of food processing in space." *Food Technology* 48 (1994): 113.

Gosch, C. C. A., ed. *Danish Arctic Explorations: 1605 to 1620.* Vol. 2, No. 96 and 97. London: Hakluyt Society, 1897.

Gould, L. M. *Cold, The Record of An Antarctic Sledge Journey.* New York: Brewer, Warren and Putnam, 1931.

Greely, A. W. *The Attainment of the Farthest North.* London: Richard Bentley and Son, 1886.

———. *Three Years of Arctic Service. An Account of the Lady Franklin Bay Expedition of 1881–84.* London: Richard Bentley and Son, 1886.

Guttridge, L. F. *Icebound, The Jeannette Expedition's Quest for the North Pole.* Annapolis, Maryland: Naval Institute Press, 1986.

Hahn, R. G. "Expedition to Another World: Biosphere 2 Crew Completes Mission One." *Explorers Journal* 71 (1993): 161–167.

Hall, C. F. *Arctic Researches and Life Among the Esquimaux. Being the Narrative of an Expedition in Search of Sir John Franklin, in the Years 1860, 1861 and 1862.* New York: Harper and Brothers, 1865.

Hannon, L. F. *The Discoverers.* Toronto: McClelland and Stewart, Ltd., 1971.

Hansson, H. *Voyages of a Modern Viking.* London: G. Routledge and Sons, 1936.

Harrison, A. A.; Y. A. Clearwater; and C. P. McKay. *From Antarctica to Outer Space.* New York: Springer-Verlag, 1990.

Hashimoto, Y. *Marine Toxins and Other Bioactive Marine Metabolites.* Tokyo: Japan Scientific Society's Press, 1979.

Hayes, I. I. *An Arctic Boat Journey in the Autumn of 1854.* London: Richard Bentley, 1860.

———. *The Open Polar Sea. A Narrative of Discovery Towards the North Pole.* New York: Hurd and Houghton, 1867.

Haymes, E. M., and C. L. Wells, eds. "Cold Environments and Human Performance." In *Environment and Human Performance.* Champaign, Ill.: Human Kinetics Publishers, Inc., 43–68.

Hearne, S. *A Journey from Prince of Wale's Fort in Hudson's Bay to the Northern Ocean.* Rutland, Vermont: Charles E. Tuttle Co., 1795.

Herodotus. *The History,* circa 450 B.C. In *Of Herodotus, Great Books of the Western World,* edited by R. M. Hutchins. Chicago: Encyclopedia Britannica, Inc., 1982.

Hippocrates. In *On Ancient Writings,* section 3, Circa 390 B.C. of *The Great Books,* translated by Francis Adams. Chicago: University of Chicago and Encyclopedia Britannica, Inc., 1982.

Hobbs, P. V. *Ice Physics.* Oxford: Oxford University Press, 1974.

Hødnebø, F., and J. Kristjánsson, eds. *The Vikings' Discovery of America.* Oslo: J. M. Stenersens Forlag A/S, 1991.

Hooper, B., ed. *With Captain Cook in the Antarctic and Pacific. The Private Journal of James Burney.* Canberra: National Library of Australia, 1975.

Hunt, W. R. *To Stand at the Pole.* New York: Stein and Day, 1981.

Huntford, R. *Scott and Amundsen.* London: Hodder and Stoughton, 1979.

———. *Shackleton.* New York: Ballantine Books, 1985.

———. *The Last Place on Earth.* London: Pan Books Ltd., 1985.

Huxley, L. *Scott's Last Expedition.* Vol. 1 and 2. London: John Murray Publishers, Ltd., 1913.

Jacka, F., and E. Jacka, eds. *Mawson's Antarctic Diaries.* London: Unwin and Hyman, 1988.

Johnson, R. E. "By Want Beleaguered: Sir Franklin (1786–1847) in the Canadian Arctic." In *Starving Sailors: The Influence of Nutrition upon Naval and Maritime History,* edited by J. Watt, E. J. Freeman, and W. F. Bynum. London: National Maritime Museum, 1981, 109–116.

————. "Doctors Abroad: Medicine and Nineteenth-century Arctic Exploration." In *Starving Sailors: The Influence of Nutrition upon Naval and Maritime History*, edited by J. Watt, E. J. Freeman, and W. F. Bynum. London: National Maritime Museum, 1981, 101–108.

Johnson, R. E., and R. M. Kark. *Feeding Problems in Man as Related to Environment. An Analysis of United States and Canadian Army Ration Trials and Surveys: 1941-1946.* Chicago: U.S. Army Medical Nutrition Laboratory, 1947.

Kane, E. K. *Arctic Explorations. The Second Grinnell Expedition in Search of John Franklin, 1853, 1854, 1855.* Philadelphia: Childs and Peterson, 1854.

————. *The U.S. Grinnel Expedition in Search of Sir John Franklin: A Personal Narrative.* London: Sampson Low, Son, and Co., 1854.

Kark, R. M.; R. E. Johnson; and J. S. Lewis. "Defects of Pemmican as an Emergency Ration for Infantry Troops." *War Medicine* 7 (1945): 345–352.

Klutschak, H., trans. *Overland to Starvation Cove (Als Eskimo Unterden Eskimaux),* by W. Barr. Toronto: Univ. Toronto Press, 1987.

Koettlitz, R. "Contributions to the Natural History of the Polar Bear (Ursus Maritimus, Linn.)." *Proc. Royal Physical Society* 14 (1898): 266–277.

Lamson, C. "Shipping in the Northwest Passage: A Pandora's Box." *Endeavour*, n. s. 10, 4 (1986): 167–176.

Lancet. *Feature Article* 1 (1823): 1069.

Landy, D. "Pibloktoq (Hysteria) and Inuit Nutrition: Possible Implication of Hypervitaminosis." *Soc. Sci. Med.* 21, 2 (1985): 173–185.

Lane, H. W. "Nutrition in Space: Evidence from the U.S. and the U.S.S.R." *Nutrition Reviews* 50 (1992): 3–6.

Lansing, A. *Endurance.* New York: McGraw-Hill Book Co., 1959.

"Lead Solder: Source of Body Lead in the Franklin Burials." *Nutrition Reviews* 48, 7 (1990): 292.

Lebedev, V. *Diary of a Cosmonaut: 211 Days in Space.* Translated from Russian by Gabriela Azrael. In cooperation with the Gloss Co. College Station, Texas: Phytoresource Research, Inc., 1988.

Leo, M. A., and C. S. Lieber. "Hypervitaminosis A: A Liver Lover's Lament." *Hepatology* 8, 2 (1988): 412–417.

Lewis, H. E. "Nutritional Research in the Polar Regions." *Nutrition Reviews* 21 (1963): 353–356.

————. "State of Knowledge about Scurvy in 1911." In "Medical Aspects of Polar Exploration: Sixtieth Anniversary of Scott's Last Expedition." *Proc. Royal Soc. Med.: Section of the History of Medicine* 65 (1972): 39–42.

Lindhard, J. "Health Conditions on the Danmark Expedition." *Medd. Grønland* (1913): 457–468.

Linscher, W. G., and A. J. Bergroesen. "Lipids." In *Modern Nutrition in Health and Disease*, edited by M. E. Shils and V. R. Young. Philadelphia: Lea and Feiger, 1988.

Lloyd, C. and J. L. S. Coulter. *Medicine and the Navy 1200-1900*. Vol. 3. Edinburgh and London: E.& S. Livingstone, Ltd., 1961, 1714–1815.

———. *Medicine and the Navy 1200-1900*. Vol. 4. Edinburgh and London: E&S Livingston, Ltd., 1961, 1815–1900.

Lockhert, E. E. "Antarctic Trail Pict." MS No. 89. National Archives.

Loomis, C. and M. A. Wilson. *The Story of Charles Francis Hall, Explorer*. New York: Alfred Knopf, 1971.

Lopez, B. *Arctic Dreams. Imagination and Desire in a Northern Landscape*. New York: Charles Scribner's Sons, 1986.

Lugg, D. J. "Antarctic Medicine: 1775–1975, Parts 1 and 2." *Medical Journal of Australia* 2 (1975): 295–298; 335–337.

———. "Antarctic Medicine: Isolation and a Hostile Climate Accentuate Some Common Problems." In *Antarctica*. Reader's Digest Cafriania Press, 1985.

———. "The Inner Man: The Importance of Food in Antarctica's Hostile Environment," In *Antarctica*. Reader's Digest Cafriania Press, 1985.

Lusk, G. *Nutrition*. New York: Paul B. Hueber, 1933.

Mackenzie, A. *Voyages from Montreal on the River St. Laurence through the Continent of North America to the Frozen and Pacific Oceans in the Years 1789 and 1793 with a Preliminary Account of the Rise, Progress, and Present State of the Fur Trade of that Country*. London: R. Noble, Old-Bailey, 1801.

Markham, C. R. *The Lands of Silence—A History of Arctic and Antarctic Explorations*. New York: Cambridge Univ. Press and The MacMillian Co., 1921.

Marriott, B. *Nutrient Requirement For Work in Cold and High Altitude Environments*. Washington D.C.: Institute of Medicine. National Academy of Sciences, Jan. 31– Feb. 1, 1994.

Mawson, D. *The Home of the Blizzard*. Vol. 1 and 2. Philadelphia: Lippincott Co., 1914.

———. *Mawson's Antarctic Diaries*. Edited by F. Jacka and E. Jacka. London: Unwin Hyman, 1988.

McClintock, L. *The Voyage of the 'Fox' in the Arctic Seas*. London: John Murray, 1860.

Melville, G. W. *In the Lena Delta*. New York: Houghton Mifflin and Co., 1885.

Miller, D. R., and K. C. Hayes. *Intake and Toxicity of Vitamins in Nutritional Toxicity*. Edited by J. N. Hathock. New York: Academic Press, 1981.

Milton-Thompson, G. J. "Two Hundred Years of the Sailor's Diet." In *Starving Sailors: The Influence of Nutrition upon Naval and Maritime History*, edited by J. Watt, E. J. Freeman, and W. F. Bynum. London: National Maritime Museum, 1981.

Moore, T. *Vitamin A*. Amsterdam: Elsevier, 1957.

Morris, C., ed. *Finding The North Pole*. New York: Viking, 1909.

Mowat, F. *Ordeal by Ice*. Toronto: McClellend and Stewart, Ltd., 1960.

———. *The Polar Passion*. Boston: Little, Brown & Co., 1967.

————. *Tundra. Selection from the Great Accounts of Arctic Land.* Toronto: McClelland and Stewart, 1973.

Nansen, F. *Eskimo Life.* London: Longmans, Green and Co., 1893.

————. *Farthest North.* New York: Harper and Brothers, 1898.

————. *The First Crossing of Greenland.* London: Longmans, Green and Co., 1892.

Nares, G. S. *Narrative of a Voyage to the Polar Sea During 1875–1876 in H.M. Ships 'Alert' and 'Discovery'.* Vol. 1 and 2, 4th edition. London: Sampson Low, Marston, Searle and Rivington, 1878.

NASA Facts. Space Shuttle Food Systems. NF150/1–86. *U.S. National Aeronautics and Space Administration,* 1986.

NASA Facts. "Food for Space Flight." NP-1996-07-007JSC. *U.S. National Aeronautics and Space Administration,* July 1996.

Neatby, L. H. "History of Hudson Bay." In *Science, History and Hudson Bay, Ottawa,* edited by C. S. Beals. Vol. 1.Ottawa: Department of Energy Mines and Resources, 1968.

————. *The Search for Franklin.* New York: Walker and Co., 1970.

Neider, C. *Edge of the World. Ross Island, Antarctica.* Garden City, New York: Doubleday and Co., 1974.

Newman, P. C. *Company of Adventurers.* Ontario, Canada: Penguin Books, Canada, Ltd., Markham, 1986.

O'Hara, W. J.; C. Allen; and R. J. Shepard. "Loss of Body Fat During An Arctic Winter Expedition." *Canadian Journal of Physiological Pharmacology* 55 (1977): 1235–1241.

O'Meara, J. J. *The Voyage of Saint Brendan: Journey to the Promised Land.* Atlantic Highlands, N.J.: Humanities Press, 1976.

Palmer, Roy, ed. *The Oxford of Sea Songs.* Oxford: Oxford Univ. Press, 1986.

Parry, W. E. *Journal of a Second Voyage ... in 1821–23.* New York: Harper & Brothers, 1824.

————. *Journal of a Third Voyage ... in 1824–25.* New York: Harper & Brothers, 1826.

————. *Narrative of an Attempt to Reach the North Pole ... in 1827.* New York: Harper & Brothers, 1828.

————. *Three Voyages for the Discovery of the Northwest Passage ... in 1819–20.* New York: Harper & Brothers, 1821.

Pasteur, L. "Method pour previnir la rage apres morsure." *Comptes Rendues de l'Academie de Sciences* 101 (1885): 765–774.

Patton, J. F., and J. A. Vogel. "Effects of Cold Exposure on Submaximal Endurance Performance." *Med. Sci. Sports, Exerc* 16 (1984): 494–497.

Peary, J. D. *My Antarctic Journal: A Year Among the Ice Fields and Eskimoes.* New York: Contemporary Publ. Co., 1894.

Peary, R. E. *The North Pole*. New York: F. A. Stokes, 1910.

———. *Northward Over the Great Ice*. New York: F. A. Stokes, 1898.

———. *Secrets of Polar Travel*. New York: The Century Co., 1917.

———. "Brief Outline of a Project for Determining the Northern Limit of Greenland, Overland: Civil Engineer USN." May 10, 1890. National Archives.

Phinney, S. D.; B. R. Bistram; W. J. Evans; E. Gervino; and G. L. Blackburn. "The Human Response to Chronic Ketosis without Caloric Restrictions: Preservation of Submaximal Exercise Capabilities with Reduced Carbohydrate Oxidation." *Metabolism* 32, 8 (1983): 769.

Pigafetta, A. *Magellan's Voyage Around the World*. Cleveland: The Arthur H. Clark Company, 1906.

Ponting, H. G. *The Great White South: or With Scott in the Antarctic*. London: Gerald Duckworth and Co., Ltd., 1922.

Priestley, R. E. "Inexpressible Island." *Nutrition Today* 4 (1969): 18–27.

Pugh, L.G.C. "The Logistics of the Polar Journeys of Scott, Shackleton and Amundsen." Part of "Medical Aspects of Polar Exploration: Sixtieth Anniversary of Scott's Last Expedition." *Proc. Royal Soc. Med., Section of the History of Medicine* 65 (1972): 42–47.

Pyne, S. J. *The Ice*. Iowa City, Iowa: University of Iowa Press, 1986.

Radok, U. "The Antarctic Ice." *Sci. American* 253, 2 (1985): 98–105.

Ralling, C. *Shackleton*. London: British Broadcasting Corp., 1983.

Rawlins, D. *Peary at the North Pole. Fact or Fiction?* Washington, D.C.: Robert B. Luce, 1973.

Read, P. P. *Alive: The Story of Andes Survivors*. Philadelphia and New York: J. B. Lippincot Co., 1974.

Reuther, R. T. "First President of the Explorers' Club—Major General Aldophus Washington Greely." *The Explorers Journal* 72, 1 (1994): 4–9.

Rich, E. E.; A. M. Johnson; J. M. Wordie; and R. J. Cyriax. *John Rae's Correspondence with the Hudson's Bay Company on Arctic Exploration*. London: The Hudson's Bay Record Society, 1953.

Richardson, J. *Polar Regions*. Edinborough: A. & B. Black, 1861.

Rink, H. *The Eskimo Tribes. Their Distribution and Characteristics, Especially in regard to Language*. New York: AMS Press, 1887–1891.

Rodahl, R., and T. Moore. "The vitamin A content and toxicity of bear and seal liver." *Biochem. J.* 37 (1943): 166–168.

Rogers, A. F. "The Death of Chief Petty Officer Evans." *The Practitioner* 212 (1974): 570–580

———. "The Influence of Diet in Scott's Last Expedition." In *Starving Sailors: The Influence of Nutrition upon Naval and Maritime History*, edited by J. Watt, E. J. Freeman, and W. F. Bynum. London: National Maritime Museum, 1981, 163–173.

Ross, J. *Narrative of a Second Voyage in Search of North-West Passage and a Residence in the Arctic Regions During the Years 1829, 1830, 1831, 1832, 1833*. London: A. W. Webster, 1835.

Sacramento Bee, July 19, 1987.

Savours, A., and M. Deacon. "Nutritional Aspects of the British Arctic (Nares) Expedition of 1875–76 and its Predecessors." In *Starving Sailors: The Influence of Nutrition upon Naval and Maritime History*, edited by J. Watt, E. J. Freeman, and W. F. Bynum. London: National Maritime Museum, 1981, 131–162.

Schley, W. S. *Report on Greely Expedition: The Greely Arctic Expedition as Fully Narrated by Lt. Greely, USA, and Other Survivors. Commander Schley's Report*. Philadelphia: Barclay and Co., 1884.

Scott, R. F. *The Voyage of the Discovery*. London: John Murray, 1905.

Shackleton, E. *The Heart of the Antarctic*. Philadelphia: B. Lippincott, 1914.

———. *South*. New York: MacMillan, 1920.

Shapley, D. *The Seventh Continent. Antarctica in a Resource Age*. Washington, D.C.: Resources for the Future, 1985.

Shearman, D. J. "Vitamin A and Sir Douglas Mawson." *British Medical Journal* 1 (1978): 283–285.

Shepard, R. J. "Adaption to Exercise in the Cold." *Sports Medicine* 2 (1985) 59–71.

Shills, M. E., and V. R. Young. *Modern Nutrition in Health and Disease*, seventh edition. Philadelphia: Lea and Febiger, 1988.

Short, I., and B. Merrilees, ed. *The Anglo–Norman Voyage of St. Brendan*, by Benedeit. Manchester: Manchester University Press, 1979.

Silverman, J. *Roll and Go, Songs of American Sailormen*. New York: Norton and Co., 1964.

Simmonns, P. L. *Sir John Franklin and the Arctic Regions*. Buffalo, N.Y.: S. H. Derby and Co., 1852.

Southcott, R. V.; N. J. Chesterfield; and D. J. Lugg. "Vitamin A Content of the Livers of Huskies and Some Seals from Antarctic and Subantarctic Regions." *Medical Journal of Australia* 1 (1971): 311–313.

Stefansson, V. *The Fat of the Land*. New York: Macmillan Co., 1956.

———. *The Friendly Arctic*. New York: Macmillan Co., 1944.

———. *Hunters of the Great North*. New York: Harcourt, Brace and Co., 1922.

———. *My Life with the Eskimo*. New York: Macmillan Co., 1927.

———. *Not By Bread Alone*. New York: Macmillan Co., 1946.

———. "The Stefansson-Anderson Arctic Expedition of the American Expedition of the American Museum: Preliminary Ethnological Report." In *Anthropological Papers of the American Museum of Natural History*, Vol. 14, (Stefansson-Anderson Arctic Expedition). New York: American Museum of Natural History, 1919.

———. *Unsolved Mysteries of the Arctic*. 1938. Reprint, New York: Macmillan Co., 1972.

Steger, W., and P. Schurke. *North to the Pole*. New York: Ivy Books, 1987.

Stewart, G. F., and M. A. Amerine. "Evolution of food processing." In *Introduction to Food Science and Technology*. New York: Academic Press, 1973.

Stewart, G. R. *Ordeal by Hunger: The Story of the Donner Party*. New York: H. Holt and Company, 1936.

Takahashi, K.; Z. Nakamiya; K. Kawakami; and T. Kitasato. "On the Physical and Chemical Properties of Biosterin (a name given to fat-soluble A) and on its physiological significance." *Scientific Papers of the Institute of Physical and Chemical Research, Tokyo* 3 (1925): 81–146.

Tannahill, R. *Food in History*. New York: Stein and Day, 1973.

Tauber, G. "Biosphere 2 Gets New Lease on Life From Research Plan," *Science* 267 (13 January 1995): 169.

Thorne, S. *The History of Food Preservation*. Kirkby Lonsdale, Cumbria, England: Parthenon Publication Group, 1986.

Todd, A. L. *Abandoned*. New York: McGraw-Hill, 1961.

Tremor, J. W., and R. D. MacElroy. *Report of the First Planning Workshop for CELSS Flight Experimentation*. NASA Conference Publication 10020. U.S. National Aeronautics and Space Administration, 1988.

Tyndal, J. *The Forms of Water in Clouds and Rivers, Ice and Glaciers*. New York: D. Appleton and Co., 1896.

U.S. Department of State. See Bauernfeind, J. C.

Vaughn, D. A. "Adaptation to austere diets." In *Symposium in Arctic Biology and Medicine, V. Nutritional Requirements for Survival in the Cold and at Altitude*, edited by L. Vaughn. Ft. Wainwright, Alaska: Arctic Aeromedical Laboratory, 1965.

Walford, R. L. "A Scientist Reflects on His '21st Century Odyssey' within Biosphere 2." *The Scientist* (January 21, 1994).

Walford, R. L.; S. B. Harris; and M. W. Guniun. "The Calorically Restricted Low-Fat Nutrient-Dense Diet in Biosphere 2 Significantly Lowers Blood Glucose, Total Leucocyte Count, Cholesterol, and Blood Pressure in Humans." *Proc. Natl. Acad. Sci. USA*, 89 (1992): 11533–11537.

Wallace, A. F. C. "Mental illness, biology and culture." In *Psychological Anthropology*, edited by F. L. K. Hsu. Revised Edition, Cambridge, Maine: Shenkman, 1972, 363–402.

Watt, J. "Some Consequences of Nutritional Disorders in Eighteenth-Century British Circumnavigations." In *Starving Sailors: The Influence of Nutrition upon Naval and Maritime History*, edited by J. Watt, E. J. Freeman, and W. F. Bynum. London: National Maritime Museum, 1981, 51.

Watt, J.; E. J. Freeman; and W.F. Bynum, ed. *Starving Sailors: The Influence of Nutrition upon Naval and Maritime History*. London: National Maritime Museum, 1981.

Webster's Third New International Dictionary. Springfield, Mass.: Merriam-Webster Inc., Publishers, 1993.

Wenck, P. A.; M. Baren; and S. P. Deqan. *Nutrition*. Reston, Va.: Reston Publishing Co., 1980.

Weyer, E. M. *The Eskimos. Their Environment and Folkways*. Hamden, Conn.: Archon Books, 1962.

index

about the author

Robert E. Feeney was born in Oak Park, Illinois, in 1913. He received his B.S. in chemistry in 1938 from Northwestern University and his Ph.D. in biochemistry from the University of Wisconsin, Madison, in 1941. Following a postdoctoral at Harvard Medical School, he spent three years in the U.S. Army (United States and New Guinea) and seven years at the U.S. Department of Agriculture Western Regional Laboratory, Albany, California. He was then professor of chemistry and chairman of the Department of Biochemistry and Nutrition at the University of Nebraska, Lincoln, NE, from 1953 to 1960. In 1960, he became research biochemist in the Agricultural Experimental Station and professor in the Department of Food Science and Technology at University of California, Davis. He became emeritus in 1984. His longtime area of research and teaching has been in the chemical modification of proteins with applications to proteins forming complexes, such as the iron-complexing transferrins and inhibitors of proteinases found in egg white and blood serum. These led to six trips to Antarctica and an equal number to northern areas and studies on the antifreeze proteins from polar fish.